D0341717

Growing Younger

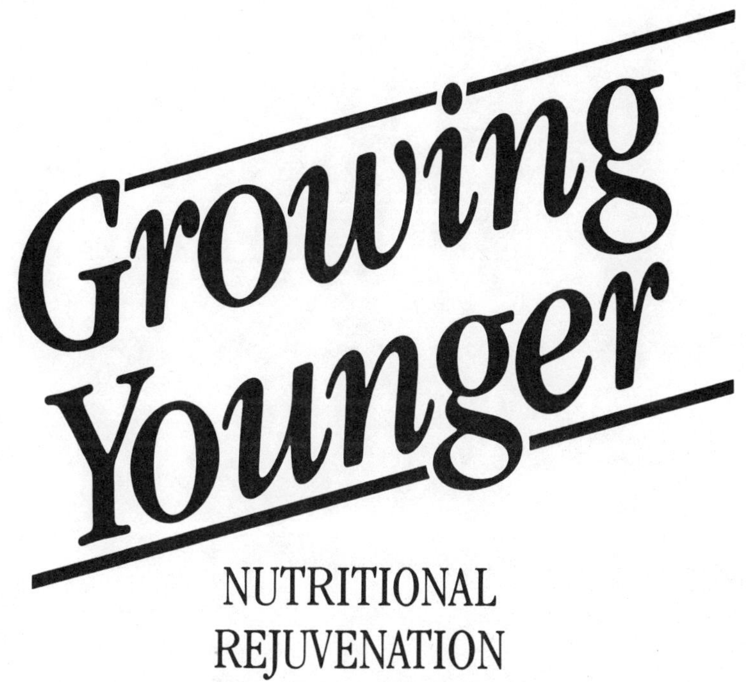

Growing Younger

NUTRITIONAL REJUVENATION FOR PEOPLE OVER FORTY

Gershon M. Lesser, M.D.

Foreword by Lee M. Shulman, Ph.D.

JEREMY P. TARCHER, INC.
Los Angeles
Distributed by St. Martin's Press
New York

Library of Congress Cataloging in Publication Data

Lesser, Gershon.
Growing younger.
Bibliography.
Includes index.
1. Health. 2. Rejuvenation. 3. Longevity. I. Title.
RA776.75.L47 1987 613 87-10004
ISBN 0-87477-434-9

Jeremy P. Tarcher, Inc.
9110 Sunset Blvd.
Los Angeles, CA 90069

Design by Mike Yazzolino

Manufactured in the United States of America

10 9 8 7 6 5 4 3 2 1

First Edition

To my wife, Michelle Elyse Lesser, whose constant companionship and encouragement allowed me to formulate the process of writing and living healthfully.

To my mother, Dora Lesser, who forever changed my medical focus when, fifteen years ago, she asked me, "Why don't you ever prescribe Vitamin A?"

Contents

PART TWO: REJUVENATION PLANS FOR SPECIFIC SYMPTOMS AND AILMENTS

Acknowledgments

I am forever indebted to my associate, Larry Strauss, who shared the entire inspiring review of this field with me, who researched untiringly and with limitless inquiry, and who in the process also taught me how to write a book. Without this man there would be no book.

I must also express my gratitude to my editor, Janice Gallagher, whose consistent, gentle, but precise literary expertise and scientific knowledge kept me always in clear and present orbit, and whose belief in the power of the individual to determine his or her own destiny catalyzed the philosophies expressed here.

Many people have helped inspire me—some have also badgered me—to write this book. In this regard I must thank all my patients, my listeners, and my professional colleagues who have appeared on my shows as guests, and I must also thank my friends: Dr. Lee Shulman, Dr. Joyce Shulman, Norman Cousins, Dr. Nathaniel Branden, Dr. Linus Pauling, Dr. Carlton Fredericks, Dr. Richard Passwater, Dr. S. Jerome Tamkin, Dr. Joel Zisk, Dr. Peter Gabor, Dr. Mark Tobenkin, Dr. Marshall Kadner, Dr. Albert Zager, Dr. Donald Rossman, Chuck Ashman, Jeff Cory, Art Linkletter, Gloria Swanson, Sally Forrest, Michael Jackson, Ruth Herschman, Will Lewis, Noel Horwin, Mitchell Harding, Tom Strothers, Robert Forst, Dick McGeary, Mike Lundy, Chuck Young, Merv Griffin, Meredith McCrae, Geoff Edwards, William Dufty, George Kostka, Paula and John Quinn, Milo Frank, Perry Polski, Sister Mary Anthony, and Father Marcos Nicholas, as well as Los Angeles County Medical Association's David Zeitlin, and Irv Atkins and Max Candiotty—agent, attorney, alter egos, and closest friends—who have been behind me all the way.

And I must thank my wife, Michelle, whose piercing questions and scientific inquiry focused my attention upon so many issues central to longevity and the good life, and whose limitless patience shared mountains of research literature strewn about our entire home—not to mention the many nearly sleepless nights shared in debating nutritional controversies.

Foreword

The ancient Greeks expressed a goal we may all aspire to, "To die young, as late in life as possible." Dr. Lesser has devoted his life to researching and disseminating ways in which we can all live young. He has made us aware of the very important connection between what goes on in our mind and spirit, and how it affects our body. And for those of us who are only vaguely aware of how our nutrition, exercise, and other habits may be affecting our lives, this man has made it his life's work to encourage us to be acutely aware.

In very clear ways he lets us know that the only way we can prolong our lives is to maintain good health habits throughout our lifetime. Prevention of disease has been his goal. He demonstrates his respect for human beings by making it clear that "health is how you choose to live your life," and that active participation is an essential part of that choice.

Dr. Lesser has been at the cutting edge of medical knowledge for the past twenty years—both in reporting the most up-to-date medical knowledge to a vast public through radio and television networks, and with breakthroughs in his own practice of prevention and treatment of illness. Although I had heard him on the Health Connection, a radio show that he has used to promote good health ideas for years, I first met him nine years ago when I began having great fatigue after one set of tennis. My wife, Joyce, told me that I looked gray, and I felt cold and clammy. I was finally motivated to see Dr. Lesser. After his initial examination, a stress test was recommended and I flunked it. With loving reassurance and encouragement, he prescribed changes in my eating habits, nutrients added to my diet, a gradual, enjoyable exercise program, and other changes in my lifestyle. I followed his prescriptions. Within a few months, a second stress test proved to be no obstacle and my youthful vigor was restored. I am a believer.

Over the years that we have known him, our admiration for him has continued to grow. We are impressed by his great depth and breadth of knowledge, his use of natural and noninvasive methods whenever possible, and his loving dispensation of all he knows and does. Megadoses of vitamin L for Love is on the wall of his office, and is his closing to each of his radio shows. It reflects his conviction that love is both physiological and psychological, and that it is the most vital nutrient of all. He teaches us that a loving nature, toward ourselves and one another, is the best prevention, and that unconditional love will transform the world. He understands the mind-body-spirit connection, and that how you look at life has everything to do with health and happiness. He knows how to talk healing talk, how to give hope, not despair, and how to encourage and support change when what you are doing isn't working for you.

The world needs the information contained in this book. It is designed to provide the data we need, with the scientific research behind each recommendation to back it up. Dr. Lesser gives us the information in a clear, accurate, and concise manner so that we can use it for life, health, and longevity. We have been gifted in our lives with many great teachers—Dr. Lesser is one of them. He teaches us how to live, not just how to cure diseases. We are deeply and profoundly honored to invite you to make this book part of your life.

LEE M. SHULMAN, PH.D.
JOYCE SHULMAN, PH.D.
Beverly Hills, California
March, 1987

A Cautionary Note

The nature of medical practice and information is flux and change, not the stability some of us may like to believe exists. More so than in almost any other science, facts and beliefs in medicine have the characteristic of never standing still. What we believe today we must be prepared to alter or discard tomorrow based on new observations. The use of leeches and ether are examples of what once were standardized practices, and while in the past it took decades, even centuries, to revise these practices, today new insights occur with the speed of light; the half-life of a medical fact in the latter part of the twentieth century is about one week.

I urge you, therefore, not to use this book as a substitute for the advice of your competent physician and counselor. My purpose in writing it is not to suggest that all is known, or that what applies to one person applies collectively to everyone.

What's good for me may be toxic for you, and vice versa. No book can know an individual as well as a physician's listening ear and searching eye. Furthermore, reasonable argument can probably present a case opposite to every suggestion made in this or any other book on healthful living. No recommendation, after all, comes without some potential for risk. Even aspirin, we now know, can cause lethal hemorrhages and ulcers in some people. My hope, then, is to interest you in seeking to take back control over your life, to show you the nature of your own self-determined longevity measure, and by doing so to involve you in seeking a better tomorrow for yourself.

I offer my observations not as a prescriptive therapy, prevention, or final word, but as a starting point for the process of thought, conversation, and investigation between you and your physician. Your excitement with the potential for prevention and self-help will grow as you further search and research the ever-growing field of nutrition, longevity, and good health.

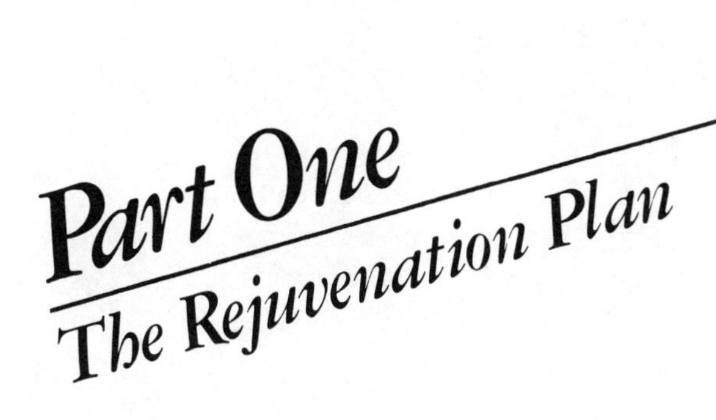
Part One
The Rejuvenation Plan

1
I Feel Better Now Than I Did at Twenty-two

What the caterpillar calls the end of the world, the master calls a butterfly.

—Richard Bach

Have you ever wondered whether you should have taken better care of your health all these years? While you were busy running a business, climbing a social ladder, raising children, or saving the world, maybe you could have been more careful about what you ate, maintained better physical fitness, and taken more time out for relaxation. Now, perhaps, a nagging sense of guilt strikes every time the doctor checks your heartbeat or draws a vial of blood with which to analyze in detail all the evidence of years of too much—or not enough—fun. Indulgence, as many of us are taught at a very early age, always catches up with us eventually. But it is not necessarily so, not if we learn the right kind of indulgence—indulging in our health. If we start right now, we don't have to pay anyone's piper.

There is no doubt about it: it is frightening to wake up

one morning and discover that you're about as old as you remember your parents being when they first began to seem old. Doctors do not always help. You have now, statistically, moved into a higher risk category for more illnesses than one cares to think about. Tests you never much thought about, or even heard of, are now advised annually or even semiannually. As a physician and cardiologist I daily see people, usually in their forties or fifties or sixties, who fear it is too late for them ever to be healthy again. Often they have no visible symptoms of anything, but they insist that they are sick. They don't feel like they used to. Life, they are sure, is a downhill slide from now on. The first bit of medical advice I give them is always that they are wrong. The human body, the most incredible machine I know of, is designed for rejuvenation, at any age.

Other patients come to me with an illness, or two or three—anything from fatigue to chronic headaches to an ulcer to the beginning of osteoporosis—and they are sure that what ails them is symptomatic of heredity and aging; their enemy, they are sure, is time. They too are wrong. It is a fascinating paradox: never before in medical history has it been so clear that deterioration and illness are, for the most part, *choices* rather than genetic inevitabilities, nor has it ever been quite so obvious what the right choices for longevity are. And yet never before have I seen so many people, in my own medical practice, so fearful of aging and illness. If my patients are any kind of representation of the general population, all of whom are extremely fortunate to be alive in a time when such choices are available, then this message needs to find many ears.

As we grow older it is junk food, cigarette smoking, alcohol abuse, stress, obesity, and lack of exercise—not Big Ben—that wears down organ systems and diminishes immunity. Aging is determined by how we choose or don't choose to live our lives. Getting well, growing younger, and rejuvenating our organ systems—not to mention our spirit—is very much within our control once we realize it and become aware of the not-so-secret secrets of rejuvenation and longevity.

There are two prominent ways in which we get sick, both well within our control: abuse of our bodies (which can be misuse or lack of use), and immune deficiency. And there are three very direct ways in which our choices affect those causes of illness and our life expectancy: through diet (which includes nutritional supplementation and the nutritional effects of medicines), exercise, and attitude.

For example, heart disease, in an overwhelming majority of cases, is a body-abuse phenomenon that can be traced to improper diet, lack of exercise, and undealt-with negative emotions. It is for most of us, therefore, a choice. Even if you're forty-five years old with high blood pressure, high cholesterol, and two brothers who died of coronaries, it is still, right now, a choice! Other abuse or lack of use choices are chronic indigestion, insomnia, ulcers, obesity, muscle aches, and various general pains. If you've read this far, you may never again be able to feel helpless and victimized.

Immune deficiency illnesses range from common colds to herpes to AIDS and cancer. And as science continues to study the aging process, more and more findings link both deterioration and rejuvenation to the immune system. One key factor is the presence of so-called "free radicals," which are bits of broken molecules in our bodies that attack and destroy cells, causing the degeneration of aging. Recent findings have indicated the immune system as the means by which we can stop these free radicals. A healthy immune system is also imperative in protecting us from cancer and viruses, which can age us. Moreover, a suppressed immunity not only leaves us vulnerable but can actually become a potential instigator of autoimmune diseases that age us. Fortunately, it is becoming increasingly clear that immunity, strong or weak, is a choice; it is the result of an action. In exploring this exciting phenomenon we shall discover some of the reasons why.

THE KEY TO GROWING YOUNGER: A STRONG IMMUNE SYSTEM

Most of us grow up believing that all sickness and cures come from outside of us. The medical profession once believed this as well. Now we know better. Prevention and cure of almost all diseases, as well as the very model of inspiration for every external medical treatment, comes primarily from within us. Immunity is not just a buzzword. It is, in the era of AIDS, herpes, and cancer, *the* medical issue of our time; and it is the continued understanding of this incredible, almost magical system, which medical science is just beginning to understand, from which flow our most pragmatic approaches to making our bodies healthier places in which to live.

When I refer to the human immune system, I am talking about the most herculean defense, the only real protection we have against bacteria, viruses, fungi, toxic chemicals, cancers, and autoimmune diseases such as rheumatoid arthritis and lupus erythematosus.

Our first line of defense is our skin, which manages to keep most unfriendly invaders out. Next comes our gastrointestinal tract, which, if it is healthy, only the most stubborn invaders can penetrate. Beyond that there are over a trillion white blood cells, each highly specialized, distributed throughout the body. In two blinks of an eye, we use, manufacture, and replace about one million of these white blood cells, all of which have but one mission in life: to search out, seize, and destroy anything that is not normal and/or friendly to the body. Such "enemies" (pathogens) include bacteria, viruses, and even our own cells if they change a little from the norm so as to become malignant.

These protective blood cells are known as *macrophages*, *lymphocytes*, and cells produced in the thymus gland called *T-cells*. In addition to these cells, we have blood secretions called antibodies which pour out and literally cover an invader like a smoke screen, immobilizing it and giving the macrophages time to consume and destroy it before it can infect us. From the T-cells we get literally hundreds of different kinds of antiviral, anti-inflammatory, antitumor chemicals called interferons. It is now a proven fact that no virus can reproduce or spread throughout the body when in the presence of a specific interferon designed to attack that particular virus. What is most amazing about this system, when it works, is that the specifically designed interferon is not produced by the thymus gland until the moment when the virus invades the body; and yet if the immune system is healthy the protective interferon seeks and destroys like a veteran combat soldier.

Without our knowing it, every day our immune system, if it is healthy, protects us from foreign invaders, including the potentially hazardous effects of polyester clothing and vapors of all kinds, ranging from synthetic carpets to leaking pilot light gas in the stove. If our immune system becomes compromised, the same pathogens that we might never have known existed can make us sick. The cancer cells, for example, that had always been rapidly destroyed in our blood stream, can now spread throughout our body. In its most extreme and tragic case, this weakened immunity is known as AIDS, not a cancer itself but an immunodeficiency that allows cancers, viruses, parasites, or other pathogens to literally consume the entire body.

The reason members of the same family or office staff or people sharing a box at the opera can be exposed to the same influenza bug yet not all get sick depends on whose immunities are working and whose are not. Pathogens are all around us, but if our white cells, lymphocytes, and T-cells are in good shape, they will not harm us.

The condition of your immune system, then, determines how healthy or sick you are. It's that simple. And it has nothing to do with age.

No one is yet certain of the totality of what causes an immunity to be strong or to be suppressed, but it is clear that without adequate zinc, iron, vitamins A, C, and E, protein, and any number of other important nutrients, and without adequate physical activity and the right outlook on life, immunity is not at all likely to be high. And we know, too, that excess alcohol, excess dietary fat, excess refined sugar, obesity, certain drugs, and stress of all kinds can and will compromise immunity. Conversely, then, a strong immunity—which all of us can have—seems to boil down to three interdependent variables: proper nutrition, consistent exercise, and healthy attitude.

And I do mean interdependent. One without the other

two is ineffective with respect to immunity and almost every other health issue. The flip side of this is that each variable of the rejuvenation lifestyle will help in the implementation of the others. Good nutrition gives us more energy, helping us in the pursuit of exercise. Exercise raises our level of the neurotransmitter serotonin and can release natural tranquilizers known as endorphins, which can help make our outlook on life a positive one. A healthy attitude of high self-esteem will not allow us to feed ourselves in an unhealthy manner, and eating the right foods will help keep us mentally vibrant. Moreover, exercise seems to moderate the appetite, putting us more in tune with what our body needs in the way of nutrition.

This is why when I see the long faces of patients who believe life for them is now in the past tense, I am so impassioned, almost desperate, to set them straight. For hopelessness, just the feeling that health and the lack of it are beyond our control, has been proven to severely suppress immunity by itself. By the same token, hope and optimism can help raise our immunity. My rejuvenation plan is long-term—at best, a lifetime—but results should begin almost immediately, provided we choose to see them. Those results can fuel us with hope, and that may prove to be the most precious of all commodities.

A PLAN OF ACTION

This is certainly not the first book intended to help you live better and longer. This means that I must be that much more persuasive in my pitch to you so that this book is the one that makes the difference, the one that inspires the kind of action that can mean living well into the twenty-first century.

The road to longevity is not always paved with clarity. There is a sometimes overwhelming barrage of current facts and theories, and frequent ambiguity. Today's "miracle food" becomes tomorrow's poison. But I have sifted through the morass to construct a common-sense approach to eating and living for health and longevity. In the first half of this book I have devoted chapters to diet, to nutritional supplements and the effects of common medications on nutrition, and a chapter each to exercise and attitude. As you will see, there is hardly a single health problem which cannot be prevented by attention to one, two, or all of these factors. For those of you who already have health problems, the second half of the book provides you with specific recommendations for treating, reversing, or preventing the recurrence of thirty-three of the most common health problems of anyone over forty.

Nothing I will suggest in these pages is particularly elaborate. It shouldn't be. My hope is that I can influence you to consider what follows as a lifetime plan, and so it offers a lifestyle choice, not a quick fix promise or a regimented system of deprivation.

NO REGRETS, PLEASE

Once we begin to realize that the clock is not responsible, that our bodies, inside and outside, are a creation of our lifestyle, that it is not how *long* we've lived but simply *how* we've lived, then we can begin to take responsibility for our health. Accepting responsibility is a wonderful thing. It is the key to achieving good health. It means waking up to the fact that we can directly improve the quality and the length of our lives, and that we can do so no matter where we are in our lives. Accepting responsibility also means feeling the thrill of personal accomplishment as we experience the results of healthy living. It means being encouraged, knowing we can take good care of ourselves. Accepting responsibility may at first mean realizing that we have, until now, done damage to ourselves.

The philosophy of this book is to go easy, be gentle. As I have stressed throughout this chapter, and will continue to stress throughout this book, without the right attitude, good nutrition and exercise will not be very effective. Self-flagellation is not the right attitude.

I used to smoke cigarettes, from age fourteen to thirty-four. I have no regrets, only gratitude that I was able to kill the habit before it killed me. I was something of a hypocrite, a doctor telling his patients to stop smoking while blowing carbon monoxide rings in their faces. And it was realizing my own hypocrisy, overhearing my own patient say, "He's telling me to quit and he smokes like a chimney," that got me to overcome my addiction.

I forgave myself. I allowed myself to be human. Being human means being imperfect. It also means being able to grow, to change, and to forgive.

We do not have to hate ourselves in order to change ourselves. We have to love ourselves.

2

The Rejuvenation Diet

Like most aspects of good health and good living, food selection can be approached from two symmetrical poles. There is no doubt now that what we choose to eat has a profound effect on the way we look and feel, inside and out. I have noticed now for quite some time that every week the pages of even the most conservative medical journals grow more and more crowded with observations and discoveries linking causes, cures, and preventions of countless diseases with diet. For some of my patients, this information is depressing. It means, they say, that more of their favorite foods are going to make them ill, or that they must deprive themselves and live a life of austerity just to live longer. For others, however, this news offers an opportunity to control their destiny, to decide for themselves how long they will live and how fit they will be. Admittedly, it may be scary to think that most of us might have to be responsible for our state of health and our state of longevity. Ultimately, however, responsibility taken seriously can lead to a new and great kind of freedom—the freedom of knowing that we can, by making the right food choices on a consistent basis, live well into the twenty-first century.

For most of us, let's face it, our eating habits are influenced most heavily by clothing size and mirror images. We walk a tightrope between culinary indulgence and a good figure, eating for looks instead of health, often jeopardizing good health and longevity in the process. But good health and good looks need not be mutually exclusive. If looking good is important to you—and why shouldn't it be?—then here's a most persuasive argument to start treating your body to a healthy intake: lasting beauty can only really be achieved from the inside out. Good health does not begin in a dress shop or at a pants rack. It begins with a choice, a single choice, about what to eat. It continues as we make additional choices to fuel ourselves with foods that will help us live longer and healthier.

Choice is a key word because we live in a society which provides us with easy access to foods that can strengthen us, as well as foods that can, over time, destroy our immune system and ultimately kill us. If we lived in the Ural Mountains of Russia and existed on tabbouli (a cracked-wheat salad) and black bread, actively farming our own food, we could grow to be 100 to 120 years old without needing to learn good nutrition. But we are living amidst a circus of junk foods, as well as nonfoods. Walk down the aisles of any supermarket, consider how much actual food surrounds you, and you'll realize a major reason why 75 percent of Americans over forty are simultaneously suffering from being overweight and malnourished. I once read the label of a nationally advertised diet product and found that it had not a single natural organic substance in it; the entire mess was conceived in laboratories. Like sleuths of good nutrition, we must seek out what is good fuel and thrive on it.

Determining what is good fuel is no simple matter. The

information on nutrition is immense and full of contradictions: polyunsaturated oils versus monounsaturated oils, for example, or claims that coffee cures asthma against evidence that coffee causes cancer and heart troubles. Carbohydrates, it seems, are not the only complex part of nutrition these days.

The Rejuvenation Diet cuts through the ambiguity and confusion so that you won't have to spend half your life trying to prolong your life. My plan is based on what I have learned from my own medical practice, which focuses on preventive medicine, inspired by what I have learned from studying the diets of those human societies who experience the highest rates of mortality and the lowest rates of heart disease and cancer. It involves nothing unique, just good bodily and nutritional care. The bottom line of almost everything I suggest is this: for real health we need real food.

This may not be a new concept for you. You may already have heard about the merits of whole, unprocessed, natural foods, and these claims may have seemed easy to dismiss. What makes this diet different, aside from the fact that it thoroughly updates the subject, is that you are about to be told to fuel yourself in a loving manner by a medical doctor, by a physician and internist who has, for twenty-three years, treated coronary thrombosis, angina, congestive heart failure, cancer, infections, hypertension, kidney failure, gallbladder disease, ulcers, colitis, strokes, diabetes, arthritis, skin disorders of all kinds, asthma, allergic diseases, irritable bowel syndrome and other digestive disorders, and who has discovered that 85 percent of all these health problems can be prevented, and most of them reversed, if we are good to ourselves nutritionally, and provided that we exercise and attain a healthy mental outlook.

Rather than thinking of the Rejuvenation Diet as a *diet* in the sense of a food prescription aimed at curing a particular disease or losing weight, let's look at the word *diet* for its primary meaning: food considered in terms of its quality, composition, and effects on health. What I am urging here is simply a change. For some perhaps it will be a slight change, for others a vast reorientation in lifestyle and eating habits to ensure good health and longevity. Nothing I recommend is meant to be temporary deprivation. Nor do I intend to make eating a miserable bore for anyone. Eating can remain a joy. What we have to do is learn to enjoy different foods and to attain a larger share of personal pleasure from the feelings that accompany a healthy diet—rather than from the smooth sedation of a chocolate cheesecake.

This may not sound revolutionary, but it is. Through eating the kinds of foods our bodies deserve we can eliminate—not just modify or cut down on but *eliminate*—heart disease. With the exception of congenital heart abnormalities, which are hereditary and quite rare, we now know that *no one else ever has to die of a heart attack.* We may also, through feeding ourselves with good fuel, improve our immunity and avoid diabetes, high blood pressure, strokes, and deterioration of muscles, tissues, and all brain functions. Moreover, we can probably rid ourselves of most cancers. And as we grow healthier inside, reversing all that ails us and beginning to grow older younger, our bodies will not only feel better, they will look better, perhaps even satisfying our scrutiny in the bathroom mirror.

GOOD FUEL/BAD FUEL

Fuel is not a hamburger with french fries and a cola. Nor is it steak and eggs with buttered toast. Fuel, as our bodies know it and use it, boils down to these molecular compounds: real (nonmanufactured) proteins, natural essential fats, complex carbohydrates, minerals, vitamins, and a mix of fibers. All of these enter us from a variety of sources. Our bodies use these substances to derive energy, to maintain proper elimination, and for the important function of restructuring ourselves. Red blood cells, for example, are replaced every 120 days; we wear two to three different sets of skin per year; and while some cells, such as brain cells, are believed never to be replaced, others, like the cells that make up the liver, die and are replaced by fresh cells every day. We are, in a sense, living inside a body much of which did not exist six months ago. It is no wonder, then, that by living on good fuel we can rejuvenate ourselves.

Flavor does not indicate the quality, or even the existence, of good fuel in a given food substance. Flavor can be created in a laboratory without containing a single natural food molecule. Texture can also be imitated. Other high-flavor, high-texture foods, such as the hamburger, fries, and cola, or the bacon, eggs, and buttered toast, contain very little good fuel in relation to harmful substances. Such foods are, quite simply, bad fuel. The nutrients they provide are far outweighed by the adverse short- and long-term effects of the fat, paste, salt, and artificial chemistry.

Separating those foods which are good fuels from those which are bad involves a variety of factors. What we want to avoid are foods high in calories, containing saturated fats (which is to say also high in cholesterol), added sodium, refined sugars and refined carbohydrates, caffeine, and chemical additives. What we want to consume, in the most imaginative, exciting, and satisfying way possible, are foods high in fiber, containing moderate amounts of monounsaturated fats, natural sugars, and high in nutrient density (meaning every calorie packed with nutrients). Since most of us are currently a part of the malnourished majority, taking destructive eating somewhat for granted, it is easiest, in distinguishing between good and bad fuels, to begin with the totality of foods and carve away the bad, leaving a beautiful, well-rounded statue of a diet. So first I will tell you what to avoid and how to avoid it, and then describe our remaining rejuvenation foods and how to make our relationship with them a fulfilling one.

Bad Fats

Fats of any kind in excess are bad fats. Dietary fat is the type of fuel that most easily turns to fat in the body, and is therefore the most common cause of obesity and all its accompanying illnesses. This is true not only because fats are the most calorie-dense of all foods (100 calories per ounce) but because they are metabolized into fat using far less energy than our bodies use to metabolize carbohydrates or proteins into fat.

Polyunsaturated fats such as corn and other vegetable oils are still considered relatively safe in moderation. This would be about one to two ounces per day. In excess, however, they are a bad fat. Excess polyunsaturates in the body are converted into what is known as arachidonic acid, which is now associated with diminished immunity and linked to certain forms of arthritis, backaches, and muscle aches. There has also been a possible link found between excess polyunsaturated fats and certain cancers. This may seem a jolting revelation in view of those not-so-long-ago claims that such oils are safe and healthy. What it underscores more than anything are two nutritional realities: theories change but excess is always a dangerous game. Furthermore, polyunsaturated fats—or, for that matter, even monounsaturated fats (which, as I will later discuss, are not only safe but beneficial to us)—are no longer safe once they are heated. Any oil, once heated, becomes hydrogenated or oxygenated, which solidifies it and turns into the kind of fat we want to avoid whenever possible: saturated fat.

To understand the dangers of saturated fats requires a brief discussion of cholesterol. There are two main types of cholesterol: *low density lipoproteins (LDL)* and *high density lipoproteins (HDL).* HDLs are an essential fatty substance responsible for carrying away cholesterol and fat from the artery wall to the liver, where cholesterol is removed through bile into the intestinal tract. HDLs are therefore needed for the prevention of arteriosclerosis and heart disease, but HDLs are produced only inside the body, and the only way we can increase this "good guy" cholesterol is through vigorous exercise. The other kind of cholesterol, LDL—"bad guy" cholesterol—is the kind you have all been warned about. It turns to sludge in the body, then combines with calcium to form and transport plaque which, over time, clogs blood vessels and causes heart attacks. The major source of LDL cholesterol in the body comes directly from the consumption of animal fats such as beef tallow and other animal lard, butter and milk fat, and egg yolks. Other saturated fats, however, when consumed are converted in the body into LDL cholesterol and are thus equally dangerous. These include tropical oils such as palm kernel oil and coconut oil, and any and all hydrogenated oils we buy or produce ourselves by frying foods in oil. In addition, these saturated fats are now known to suppress immunity, to cause ulcers as well as stomach and bowel problems, and they are now heavily linked to a variety of cancers. In Holland, for example, where the average diet contains the most saturated fat of any diet anywhere in the world, Dutch women have the highest rate of breast cancer and Dutch men have the highest rate of prostate cancer. The United States, incidentally, is a close second in saturated fat consumption and cancer risk.

The **First Goal** of our rejuvenation diet is therefore to decrease our consumption of saturated fats to *no more than 10 percent of total caloric consumption,* and preferably less. At the risk of being obvious, here are some tips. Avoid fried foods. Frying not only soaks food with saturated fat but also annihilates nutrients. Avoid red meats (with the possible exception of lean flank steak and dry leg of lamb), chicken and turkey skins, butter, whole milk (the most common American source of saturated fat and cholesterol) and whole milk products such as cream, ice cream, and solid or creamed cheeses. Avoid eggs as much as possible, since one egg contains 300 milligrams of cholesterol, which is all the average person can consume per day without raising LDL cholesterol levels above safe limits. Not so obvious, however, are the saturated fats contained in most processed or junk foods. Potato and other chips, and frozen breaded chicken or fish are loaded with these dangerous oils. So are many breakfast cereals, especially the heavy granola style, often ironically catagorized as a "health" food. Most all baked goods are made with shortening, most of them consisting of saturated fats. Delicatessen-style luncheon meats (even some claiming to be low in fat) contain more saturated fats than we can afford to play around with. Finally, perhaps the most deceptively hidden saturated fats of all are contained in certain commercial shortenings whose labels claim they contain "100% vegetable oil," while a close reading of the label shows that two of those "vegetable" oils are the dreaded palm kernel and coconut. We must read labels, sometimes, to protect ourselves; but the safest way to avoid hidden bad fats is simply to avoid processed foods. And doing so will make it easier to avoid the second major dietary health threat.

Salt: Too Much of a Good Thing

Like most other minerals, sodium is crucial to our bodies. It maintains the balance of our fluids, keeping us from dehydration, switches on and off key hormones in our body, and helps the heart, kidneys, and adrenal glands to monitor all our bodily functions. Salt maintains an adequate blood pressure and is needed by our body's electrical system.

Too much salt, however, can be deadly. Salt causes the body to retain water, and an excess of salt in the body floods the system with two to four extra quarts of fluid. Since the body is a closed system—that is, we cannot construct extra blood vessels to hold the additional fluid—this puts a tremendous strain on the heart, which now has to work twice as hard to pump all this fluid around. Too much salt can also cause kidney damage and a host of other complications.

The average American, probably without realizing it, ingests 10,000 to 14,000 milligrams of sodium per day. The **Second Goal** of our Rejuvenation Diet is to cut that intake to no more than 1000 milligrams per 1000 calories; this comes to between 1500 to 3000 milligrams of sodium per day. Merely keeping the salt shaker out of our hands isn't enough to keep our sodium at safe levels. One teaspoon of baking soda contains more sodium than a teaspoon of table salt! Smoked, cured, and in any way processed meats are soaked with salt (even those boasting "low sodium" contain more salt than is good for us), as are other processed foods, including dressings, frozen and canned foods, vegetable juices, soy sauce, and club soda. Even ice cream, baked goods, and cookies all contain incredible amounts of salt. In fact, apple pie contains more salt per ounce than french fries. The reason apple pie does not taste salty is that it contains an even more frightening amount of refined sugar and other anesthetizing—and cost saving—sweeteners. Many over-the-counter medications also contain sodium, as do some vitamin and mineral tablets. Avoiding excess salt means reading labels. It also means not replacing salt with any of the new commercial "salt substitutes" which are high in potassium and can endanger our heart rhythms.

Salt occurs naturally in every food, and it is those natural salts that we want—*nothing more.* If we buy food in its fresh, wholesome state, we do not need to employ the preservative talents of sodium chloride. If we are truly imaginative in our kitchens, there are many ways to enhance the flavor of food without adding salt. Some examples: all spices not containing salt are safe and should be encouraged, the hotter the better; my favorites are ginger root, fresh ground black pepper, and paprika. Other unsalted and exciting seasonings include garlic, onion, mustard, lemon, unsalted nuts and seeds, oranges and other fruits, pureed vegetables and vegetable juices, red peppers, jalepeño peppers, radish and horseradish, rice malt, and rice vinegar. Cooking with wine or sherry also adds flavor without salt.

If we give our taste buds a chance to taste the natural salts that exist in all foods, they may after a short while satisfy our flavor needs. And as we retrain our taste buds to appreciate subtlety and abhor overkill, we might even lose our craving for the third nutritional offender.

The Overkill Food: Refined Carbohydrates

Simple or refined carbohydrates—the various forms of white paste—are most commonly served to us as white sugar, white flour, white rice, and the thousands of nicely packaged pseudo-food products produced with these substances, are lacking in nutritional values while being high in calories. High in flavor intensity, refined carbohydrates create rapid food addictions, causing obesity and diabetes, lowering immunity, and greatly increasing the risk of heart disease. At the very least, they produce a variety of mood swings, from anxiety to depression, and create stress.

There are literally mountains of books and journals dealing with the dangers of refined sugars and starches, and while reading this literature may help you to feed yourself better, I can save you a lot of time with just three words: avoid refined carbohydrates. They are metabolized rapidly by the body, which dumps insulin, creating a temporary spurt of energy that is followed by a prolonged lethargy and depression. This high/low swing puts a tremendous strain on our bodies, especially the cardiovascular system. Refined sugars and starches turn quickly to fat; they do not satisfy hunger but perpetuate it, creating in many people an obesity cycle. They are also now linked to cancer, ulcers, stomach disorders of all kinds, and even vision problems. Perhaps the most devastating blow I can deliver to refined sugars and carbohydrates, though, is that when they are present in our bodies in excess, our body may turn them into cholesterol. What happens is that the sugar glycerine molecules get turned into triglycerides, which are, at the very least, a dangerous lipid; and at the very worst, the liver converts the triglycerides into cholesterol. That's right—low-fat, high-refined-sugar diets do not lower cholesterol, they raise it. Need I say more?

The **Third Goal** of our Rejuvenation Diet is thus to eliminate, or at least reduce to insignificant amounts, our intake of refined sugars and refined carbohydrates. Staying away from processed foods and nonfoods alone will keep mounds of white paste out of our bodies. Eliminating added salt will also help, as the salt shaker is one of the most common, if least suspected, places where refined sugar is hidden. As with limiting salt, once the taste buds get used to the subtlety of real flavors, as opposed to the pretentious blast of manufactured sweetness, the sweet tooth may be satisfied by the splendid sweet taste of a yam or a pear. Even dried fruit is a good healthy alternative, and for cooking, blackstrap molasses makes a great natural sweetener that is packed with nutrients: the B and E vitamins, copper, magnesium, and more calcium than milk!

Other Anti-Rejuvenation Foods to Avoid

Junk food, by its very name, indicates the self-worth of the person who attempts to live on it. Besides being the prime source of saturated fats, excess sodium, refined sugars, and refined carbohydrates, junk food is dangerous because it pretends to be real food while it is often devoid of nutrients.

Even products that start out as good nutrient-dense food, like chicken, can end up as junk food.

	Cal.	**Fat**	**Chol.**	**Sodium**
Arby's turkey sandwich	510 g	24 g	70 mgs	1220 mgs
J-in-the Box cheeseburger	628	35	110	1666
Kent Fried Chick (1 piece)	343	23	109	549
McDs—Egg McMuffin	327	14.8	229	585
McDs—Big Mac	563	33	86	1010

FAST FOOD NUTRITIONAL INFORMATION

Some of these fast food empires have recently begun advertising in health magazines, claiming their product is "natural" (a word without a legal definition) and health-promoting; but I don't notice them confessing to any of the preceding statistics.

There are other kinds of junk that should be kept out of our bodies because it often contains artificial chemicals and "drugs" which are harmful to us. The most pervasive of the latter is caffeine. It is no secret that caffeine is an addictive drug causing anxiety, stress, and insomnia. Now, as cited last year in the *New England Journal of Medicine,* there is a direct link between drinking coffee and coronary heart disease. Many in the medical profession are beginning to see a strong association between coffee and headache, and between coffee and cancer. And yet it is still the most abused chemical in our country. Caffeine is most prevalent in coffee. One cup of brewed coffee dumps 100 to 150 milligrams of caffeine into your bloodstream. Instant coffee has 90 to 160 milligrams per cup. Amaretto, cappuccino, and Swiss mocha contain from 40 to 76 milligrams per cup; decaf coffees can range from 3 to 15 milligrams per cup, depending on the quality of the beans they use. (Most coffee manufacturers tend to use the cheaper beans to make their decaf, which ironically contain the most caffeine.) Other beverages containing caffeine are tea (60 to 80 milligrams per cup), cola (30 to 60 milligrams caffeine per 12 ounces), other phosphorus drinks such as Mountain Dew and Dr. Pepper (54 and 40 milligrams per can, respectively), and cocoa (15 to 40 milligrams per cup). Chocolate of any kind contains caffeine (6 milligrams per ounce) as do many medicines, for example: Anacin and Midol (64 milligrams caffeine per recommended dosage), Excedrin (130 milligrams per dose), and the so-called weight control pill Dexatrim contain a 200-milligram blast of caffeine per swallow. Needless to say, any realistic rejuvenation diet cannot possibly tolerate the regular use of caffeine (or any other harsh stimulant for that matter).

Here is the **Fourth Goal** of our Rejuvenation Diet: if you are an occasional user of caffeine, become a very occasional user. Or, why not become a former user of caffeine right away? If you haven't yet developed an addiction to this highly addictive chemical, consider yourself fortunate and quit altogether. If you are already addicted to coffee or other substances high in caffeine, cutting down will help; but ultimately, if you are serious about growing younger, caffeine simply can no longer be a regular part of your life. What I recommend for my patients with caffeine addictions is to level off in a stepwise fashion down to zero. You might try using one of the 100% cereal-grain coffee substitutes, such as Pero or Linden tea. But do not quit coffee cold turkey; caffeine withdrawals are at the least unpleasant, and potentially dangerous. For further tips on detoxing from this and other addictions, I suggest Doctor Phyllis Saifer's and Merla Zellerbach's book, *Detox*.

If I haven't convinced you yet to give up coffee, chocolate, and cola beverages, there are additional hazards connected with them. Coffee, for example, contains a high dose of acidity, which, first thing in the morning—or any time of day—can cause any number of gastrointestinal maladies. Coffee also greatly compromises the calcium our body needs to strengthen our bones and prevent osteoporosis. In fact, every cup of coffee washes out 15 milligrams of calcium from our bodies, and we need to ingest 100 milligrams of calcium in order to replenish those 15 milligrams the cup of coffee drained away. Chocolate is high in saturated fat and usually—unless it is very bitter—accompanied by a major assault of refined sugar. Cola contains high amounts of sugar or potentially cancer-causing sweeteners, and a barrage of artificial colorings, flavorings, and other chemicals, none of which is of any use to our bodies. But, of course, such nutrient-deficient, and sometimes dangerous, chemical additives can be found in literally thousands of food items.

In 1950 the American Food and Drug Association enacted the first ban against a food additive; in that case it was an artificial sweetener called dulcin. In 1960 the root beer flavoring safrole was banned. Since then, green dye #1, violet #1, red #2, and orange B have all been kept out of our supermarkets; but there are hundreds of other chemicals still being tested (or not yet challenged), any number of which could be responsible for mutagenetic changes which could cause cancer. I am not willing to wait for the FDA to outlaw a laboratory-invented chemical before I stop putting it down my throat. I urge you not to either.

Obviously not every bottle of wine contains sulfur dioxide and not every pack of chewing gum is poisoned with BHA. A careful reading of labels can help us sort through the chemical madness; but in order to eliminate any possibility that we might consume any of these toxins in dangerous quantities, I urge you to adopt the **Fifth Goal** of our Rejuvenation Diet: avoid all processed foods whenever possible.

Drugs and alcohol abuse, I don't think I have to tell you, will compromise your health and shorten your life considerably (and this includes a certain mail order tea appearing on the market recently, which contains cocaine). Moderate use of alcohol—that is *one drink per day*—has recently been suggested to be good for our cardiovascular system, with no apparent side effects. But you can't save up your one drink per day and have seven on Sunday. Anything more than a drink a day of alcohol suppresses our immunity by decreasing our white blood cell levels, increasing susceptibility to illness. This is especially true

CHEMICAL ADDITIVES TO AVOID WHEN POSSIBLE

Chemical	Commonly found in
Blue #1	beverages, candy, baked goods
Blue #2	beverages, candy
Citrus Red #22	skin of some Florida oranges
Green #3	beverages, candy
Red #3	cherries in fruit cocktail
BVO	soft drinks
BHA	cereals, chewing gum, potato chips, vegetable oils
BHT	cereals, chewing gum, potato chips, oil
Propyl Gallate	vegetable oil, meat products, potato sticks, chicken soup base, chewing gum
Quinine	tonic water, quinine water, bitter lemons
Sodium Nitrite and Nitrate	Bacon, ham, franks, lunch meats, smoked fish, corned beef
Sulfur Dioxide (a.k.a. Sodium Bisulfite)	sliced fruit, wine, grape juice, dehydrated potatoes

if we are already sick; a couple of hot toddies will only prolong a cold or flu. Excess alcohol may even be a factor in the onset of cancer. Women who drank three or more alcoholic beverages per day were found to have a 40 percent higher risk of developing breast cancer than women who did not.

Watch out for herb teas. Many of them contain unknown compounds, leaves and roots we do not understand which can be dangerous. Rosehips, peppermint and other mints, and pretty much any herb teas put out by a major food company are safe, if only because these companies do not like to risk lawsuits; but some popular herb teas found in some health food stores and touted as promoting longevity, such as burdock root, hydrangea, and wormwood, are regularly being found by doctors to cause hallucinations in some people who drink them. Other herb teas, such as buck tea and quadgrass, may act as diuretics, depleting the body of important minerals. This drawback, however, is not at all unique to herb teas. Sodas of all kinds have the same effect; their excess phosphorus can deplete us of iron and calcium, and may be part of the cause of anemia and osteoporosis in many people. Sodas are also loaded with refined sugars and/or other dangerous chemicals.

Stay away from artificial sweeteners as well. Even if you don't believe that sodium saccharin causes cancer, there is no doubt that, like salt, if ingested in large quantities it may retain water and raise blood pressure. It also increases the appetite and can contribute to obesity. Sorbitol, an alcohol commonly used as a glucose substitute, can cause severe diarrhea, gaseousness, and indigestion. And as for the latest low-cal sweetener, aspartame is now believed to cause migraine headaches, anxiety, and other behavioral problems in some people. While most of us experience no side effects from this substance, there is yet another reason—perhaps the best reason of all—to stop sprinkling chemically manufactured sweetness onto food: we are merely feeding an addiction. If we give our taste buds a chance to relearn the taste of natural sugars that exist in all complex carbohydrates, we can come to recognize the elegance of natural flavors—and artificial food products will begin to taste metallic, phony, and inferior.

Avoiding Anti-Rejuvenation Foods: Staying Along the Sides

I used to advise my patients that the safest way to shop in a supermarket was to stay along the sides. That way they could get their fresh produce, fresh fish and seafood, and fresh, nonfat dairy, staying out of the aisles which are full of prepackaged high-fat, high-sodium, white, pasty, chemicalized foods. Then I discovered that many of the beans and peas are in the aisles, and so are the spices, the vinegar, and the monounsaturated oils. My best advice to you now is to be sensible. Let your motto be: "Only the best for my body." Maintain this attitude as much as possible, but do not insist on perfection. Nothing I suggest is meant as an ultimatum. Whatever you can accomplish will help. While I urge you never to eat another corned beef sandwich, one corned beef sandwich does not bring on a coronary. Bacon and eggs for breakfast once in a while will not clog your arteries. But giving up on this plan because you didn't eat ideally for one day, thus allowing suicidal eating habits to flourish—that, perhaps more than anything else, will quash the rejuvenating process. So please do not be overwhelmed by what I have and am about to recommend. If life would not seem worth living without an occasional ice cream cone, don't kill yourself; have your ice cream. Ice cream is less destructive than a lot of other high-fat, high-sodium, white paste foods simply because no one believes that two scoops of pistachio is a good nutritional plus, whereas those hamburgers and fries keep trying to impersonate a well-balanced meal. If you can cut your salt consumption by half, it may still be higher than I or any physician would recommend, but you're still better off than you were. The same is true of calorie consumption and fat intake, as well as the eating of refined carbohydrates. To whatever degree you can keep these degenerating items out of your body, to that degree you will begin to grow healthier. As you begin to replace them with what is to follow, however, and discover how good real food can really be, and as you begin to feel the results of good nutrition, as many of my own patients have, your desire to eat things that compromise your health will greatly diminish or cease entirely.

REAL FOODS TO LIVE ON— HOW SWEET THEY ARE

Now that we've carved away the saturated fat, the white paste, the sodium, and all the other anti-rejuvenation foods and nonfoods, what's left is a statuesque variety of whole natural foods from which we can derive all the components that can, in moderation, help us out in a state of rejuvenation. Moderation is a key concept of rejuvenation and is the first order of business, followed by the key nutritional ingredients of longevity, and the best way to get them.

The Joys of Eating Lightly

From eating too much to exercising beyond our limit to trying to accomplish too many things in too little time, excess can make even things that are good for us bad for us. Recent studies suggest one very basic principle: eating lightly increases longevity. In a Cornell University study, laboratory rats fed half as many calories (while getting sufficient nutrients) lived twice as long as their regularly fed cousins. Anthropologists studying societies boasting the longest life-span, where people commonly live well beyond one hundred years, have discovered a pervasive similarity among these people who live as far apart from one another as the Caucasus in Southern Russia, the Andes in South America, and the Hunza Valley of Pakistan: they all share a well-balanced diet that is very low (by our standards) in calories.

These masters of longevity may not understand why their small caloric intake enables them to live so long, but in studying them, Western medicine has come up with an explanation: as people get older, the metabolism slows down, the body becomes more efficient—more miles per calorie—so that it requires less fuel and must consume fewer calories in order to maintain a healthy body weight. There are theories that a weight gain with age is healthy, but they are in complete contradiction to my experience and to all the most recent medical literature on the subject by those I most respect. Middle-aged spread, in men or in women, is not a sign of wealth—not true wealth, anyway. Fat is the sign of a heart being worked too hard, and of other impending illnesses. Being too thin, in contrast, may also be dangerous. It can be an indication that inadequate nutrients are being consumed, and it can lead to an inadequate production of hormones. Being too thin can also be a symptom of other illnesses, such as malabsorption syndrome. But "too" thin is not an easy distinction. A mirror will not tell you. Only a medical examination will. We can, however, follow some general guidelines to find our approximate appropriate weight:

For women, 100 pounds for the first five feet of height plus 5 pounds for every additional inch; for men, 110 pounds for the first five feet of height plus 6 pounds for every additional inch. Any weight close to fitting these formulas is probably a good rejuvenation weight. How we achieve that is by moderating our caloric intake.

The average American over forty consumes more than 2700 calories per day. Many people swallow three to six thousand per day. This is far more fuel than our bodies need (especially if we have not been exercising regularly), and it is stored as fat. Since we do not live in fear of massive famines, or anticipate any likely food shortages, fat is an unnecessary, not to mention unhealthy, part of our lives. Eating lightly, then, is the **Sixth Goal** of our Rejuvenation Diet.

The average woman over forty needs about 1300 to 1500 calories per day (1800 to 2000 if she is very active) in order to sufficiently fuel her body. The average man requires anywhere from 2100 up to 2900 calories per day, if he is very active. No one should consume fewer than 1200 calories per day. Crash diets that recommend less are not safe and can do severe damage, such as muscle degeneration, heart disease, and death, especially as we get older.

Eating lightly does not mean skipping meals, or starvation with occasional binges, which can be extremely dangerous, causing, among other things, a rapid onset of arteriosclerotic blood vessels. Eating lightly means eating intelligently. Limiting our intake, we must make sure the calories we take in contain the nutrients our bodies need. For this reason, we want to focus our diet on the most nutrient-dense foods; that is, the foods with the most vitamins, minerals, proteins, fiber, and essential fatty acids per calorie. In doing so, we will be consuming foods that are both satisfying to the taste and filling to the stomach, making eating lightly much easier than one might anticipate.

If the idea of eating less still seems intimidating, keep reading. As I will explain in more detail later, a regular exercise program is the best known natural appetite regulator. It seems to suppress or raise the appetite to the level appropriate to maintain a healthy body weight, while increasing our capacity to burn calories, even while we are resting. If the idea of eating less still seems dreadfully unfulfilling, think of it this way: if you consume fewer calories on a permanent basis (while getting enough nutrients) and live that extra twenty or thirty or forty years, you will actually wind up getting a chance to eat more food over the course of your life than you otherwise would have.

With that in mind, on to the rejuvenation fuels!

H_2O: Our Much-Forgotten Necessity

I purposely place water at the head of our diet to emphasize its importance in the hope that you will never forget it. Without water there is no life. Every cell of our body needs water to send messages to the brain and to carry oxygen. Water is the main ingredient of our blood, and it is essential for the digestion of food and the transport of waste products out of the body.

While our thirst tends to diminish with age, this is not an indication that we need less water. In fact, we need more water now than we did ten years ago, due to a variety of factors, including the foods we eat, our lifestyle, and normal body changes over time. Probably one of the major causes of constipation and other bowel problems is lack of daily water consumption. The cure, therefore, is simple: drink more water. Ten to fourteen 8-ounce glasses a day is the **Seventh Goal** of our Rejuvenation Diet. It may sound like a tall order, but I consider it about as radical as wanting to live to be ninety or one hundred years old.

Make sure the water is good. Toxins commonly found in

tap water today are lead, pesticides (which enter the water supply through ground swells), industrial waste products such as PCB and arsenic, chlorine (intentionally added to water to kill bacteria, and which has now been found to be a carcinogen), and finally the natural parasites such as the amoeba giardia. Bottled water can sometimes be a good solution to our need for clean drinking water, but it can also be an expensive way of getting water no better than what comes out of your sink. If you buy water or plan to, find out where it comes from. There are a number of good consumer reports on bottled water which are well worth looking into. Debra Lynn Dadd's *Nontoxic & Natural* also contains an extensive section on water. If you really want to treat yourself like a friend, attach a filter to your water lines. I recommend a carbon and osmosis membrane filter. The expense is well worth that priceless commodity of good health.

Good Protein Comes in Small Packages

There is a common misconception among Americans regarding how much protein our bodies really require. Most of us eat far too much of it, primarily because the average diet and the very concept of a diet are centered around the major protein sources. Most restaurant menus list their entrees by the protein—the beef, lamb, veal, chicken, pork, and fish—whereas the vegetables, grains, and potatoes are all side dishes.

Protein does play a vital role in our diets; the lack of it can compromise our immunities and our health. Protein is the living substance of genetic programming and of our cells and their processes. We are, in part, made of protein. Eighteen percent of our body weight consists of protein, and our bodies use this protein to rebuild thousands of cells every day. If we do not consume adequate amounts of protein we will suffer from such problems as lowered immunity (giving way to infections), rapid aging of tissue, loss of libido, and degeneration of liver, heart, and kidneys. Lack of protein can also cause patchy brown spots to appear on the skin, loss of hair, and can instigate diarrhea, anemia, vitamin deficiencies, fluid retention and high blood pressure, and an onslaught of cognitive maladies: apathy, irritability, poor concentration, memory loss, and general fatigue. But too much protein is equally dangerous.

Excess protein becomes toxic in our bodies and puts a strain on the kidneys, increasing uric acid which can over time, if the genetic predisposition is there, cause gout or gouty arthritis. But most dangerous of all, too much protein equals obesity.

Proteins come in many shapes and sizes. They are composed of twenty-one building blocks called *amino acids.* Eleven of these amino acids can be produced by our own bodies; the other ten must come from our diet. Meat, fish, fowl, and dairy products contain all twenty-one of these amino acids, in the proper ratio, and are called complete proteins. Many other foods, such as vegetables and grains, contain only some of the amino acids. These are called incomplete proteins and must be combined properly to form complete proteins. Rice and beans is the most universal example of this. There are many other good examples, found in the books, *Diet For a Small Planet* by Frances M. Lappe and *Diet and Nutrition: A Wholistic Approach* by Dr. Rudolph Ballentine.

Considering the above, meat might be thought of as the simplest way to get complete protein; but, unfortunately, complete protein isn't all you are going to get out of your average slice of prime rib. Red meat is high in saturated fat. Pork is worse. Chicken and turkey, unless the skin is removed, are still far from ideal protein sources.

A healthy intake of protein is about 0.8 grams per 1 kilogram of body weight per day. To calculate this multiply your body weight, in pounds, by .36. (If, say, you weight 100 pounds your body requires 36 grams—or just under 2 ounces—of protein every day).

The **Eighth Goal** of our Rejuvenation Diet is to make protein about 12 to 15 percent of our total calories. In order to do this, we must get our protein from low-fat sources. Therefore, 40 percent of our protein intake should be from fish, nonfat dairy, and skinless poultry. The other 60 percent is best consumed through beans, other vegetables, and whole grains. To illustrate this point, here are some examples of protein sources with their protein and fat content (both measured in grams).

PROTEIN AND FAT ANALYSIS OF SOME COMMON FOODS

Protein source	Protein content	Fat content
3 oz broiled hamburger	24 g	17 g
3 oz mozzarella	21	15
3 oz tofu	8	4
1 cup brown rice	5	1
1 medium potato	4	0
3 oz water-packed tuna	21	1
⅔ cup kidney beans	8	0.5

The tuna and the kidney beans are easily the best protein sources; this is true for most all fish and legumes, which are low in fat, protein-dense, and appetite-satisfying. The above servings of tuna and beans and rice provide as much as half of our daily protein needs, without a lot of calories. And there are other great reasons to get our protein needs from these sources, as you will discover through learning the importance of essential fatty acids, fiber, nutrient density, and complex carbohydrates.

Getting the Essential Fats

Fats are a necessary part of our diet. They contain essential fatty acids which are needed to formulate hundreds of chemicals in our bodies. Essential fatty acids make up the components of our entire hormone system, so that diets which completely eliminate fats, or reduce them too drastically, can severely disrupt our hormonal basis, causing a variety of problems from frigidity in women to diminished libido in men. Essential fatty acids are needed to control prostaglandins, chemicals needed to mediate immunity and prevent inflammation, as well as lubricate our joints and form the lining of our cells. Our immune system depends upon certain fatty acids, as do the lining of our cells and our nervous system; even our brains are greatly dependent on fats.

Having eliminated or drastically reduced all saturated fats from our diet, we want to lubricate our insides with *small amounts* of these good fatty acids: linoleic acid, linolenic acid, gamma-linolenic acid, and eicosapentanoic acid (a.k.a. EPA).

The linoleic and linolenic acids are found in monounsaturated oils, such as olive oil, hybrid safflower oil, evening primrose oil, and borage (or canola) oil. They are now known to raise our immunity and actually *lower LDL cholesterol,* without lowering our helpful HDL cholesterol. We must, however, remember that they are a fat and are therefore high in calories. I have had patients and listeners hear me recommend olive oil but not listen to my warning about amounts, and then complain of gaining weight. One tablespoon per day is enough to reap the benefits without severely raising our caloric intake. Cold-pressed virgin is the best kind of olive oil, and also the most expensive, which may help you to maintain a moderate intake of it.

The gamma-linoleic acids are found in polyunsaturated oils, which come from vegetable and nut oils. They are a major precursor to prostaglandins, helping us to maintain healthy blood vessels, good brain functions, and high immunity. There is still much research to be done on prostaglandins. There appear to be some "good" ones which reduce infections, and other "bad" ones that catalyze infections, but it does not at this point seem that one can control "good" versus "bad" prostaglandins through choices in fat consumption. But in the small amounts recommended, there should be no danger. Polyunsaturated oils do not raise LDL cholesterol, but they do not lower it either. There is also evidence that excess polyunsaturates may be processed into arachidonic acids, causing muscle and body aches, especially lower back pain. Other recent studies have linked excess polyunsaturates to free radical production and increased cancer risk. There are, however, two particular polyunsaturated oils which appear to give the greatest gamma-linoleic benefits while producing the least of these side effects. They are hybrid safflower oil and sunflower seed oil. Like the monounsaturates, a little goes a long way. Our one tablespoon per day of oil should be divided between monounsaturates and these two good polyunsaturates.

Eicosapentanoic acids (which I will, from this point on, mercifully refer to as EPA) are long chain fatty acids found in fish oil as well as some vegetables and legumes (though no one is yet sure if our bodies can correctly process them from nonfish sources, thus I can only recommend them from marine sources). This oil, found in most marine fish, was discovered as the result of studies done on the Eskimos, whose diet is primarily fish, including whale blubber, and whose heart disease rate is the lowest in the world. EPA is now known to lower LDL ("bad guy") cholesterol and thus prevent arteriosclerosis and heart disease. EPA also fights arthritis, psoriasis, and a variety of inflammations; it raises our immunity and lowers blood pressure. Some doctors are even recommending EPA fish oil capsules, though they have been known to cause excessive bleeding, even increased stroke risk in some people (and must never be taken in conjunction with aspirin). This side effect, however, is not likely to happen as long as we get our EPA from food sources. Consuming our EPA directly from the fish will also decrease our chances of consuming too much of this essential fat.

The **Ninth Goal** of our Rejuvenation Diet, then, is to get 15 to 20 percent of our daily calories from monounsaturates, certain polyunsaturates, and deep-water marine fish high in EPA omega-3 (unless you have gallbladder problems, in which case *any* fat may be bad news and you should consult your physician before using any of these).

BEST MONOUNSATURATED FAT SOURCES

Olive oil

Borage or canola oil (a.k.a. rapeseed oil)

BEST POLYUNSATURATED FAT SOURCES

Hybrid safflower oil

Sunflower seed oil

BEST EPA OMEGA-3 FISH OIL SOURCES*

Mackerel

Herring

Bluefish

Salmon

Tuna

Cod

Shrimp

Flounder

Haddock

Swordfish

As you can see, our focus on fish as a protein source gives us more than just good protein. And so, you will discover, do the vegetables, legumes, and whole grains.

The Fiber Mix

There are two kinds of dietary fiber, both imperative to good health and longevity. Water-insoluble fiber, such as wheat bran, is needed the ensure good digestion and good, thorough elimination from our stomach and colon. Typical American diets, low in this kind of fiber, are a major cause of constipation and other bowel dysfunctions, inflammation of the intestines, diverticulosis, and carcinoma of the colon. Recent evidence suggests that this kind of fiber is also needed to protect against

*There are several nut sources of omega-3 as well—walnuts, butternuts, beechnuts, and grain sources, wheat germ and oat germ, as well as certain vegetables and beans—but it is still controversial as to whether our bodies are able to convert the omega-3 and use it from these sources.

other gastrointestinal disorders such as gallstones, high cholesterol, appendicitis, hemorrhoids, and hiatal hernia. Water-soluble fiber, such as oat bran and the pectin in fruits, vegetables, and legumes absorbs fat in the stomach, intestines, and blood and carries it out in the stool, thus lowering LDL ("bad guy") cholesterol. This kind of fiber also helps raise HDL ("good guy") cholesterol by helping prevent reabsorption of bile acids and cholesterol from the small intestines and by slowing the absorption of sugar.

With much medical talk in recent years about the importance of fiber, there are now a great slew of breakfast cereals claiming to be the most complete fiber sources available. Unfortunately, while some of them may contain some good water-soluble fiber, many of them also contain refined sugar and added sodium. They are, therefore, not good sources of fiber. Some of the granola-style cereals even contain saturated fat.

The **Tenth Goal** of our Rejuvenation Diet is to consume 40 to 60 grams of fiber per day, and to get it from as great a variety of natural unprocessed sources as possible. Here are the best sources of each kind of fiber:

WATER-INSOLUBLE FIBER

oat bran, wheat bran, barley, kasha (buckwheat), brown rice, potatoes, yams, carrots, all beans and peas.

WATER-SOLUBLE FIBER

oat bran, pears, apples, bananas, cantaloupes, watermelons, honeydews, kiwis, all berries, peaches, pineapple, raisins, figs, prunes, papayas, artichokes, asparagus, broccoli, Brussels sprouts, celery, carrots, cauliflower, cabbage, corn (popped or on the cob), parsley, parsnips, peppers, potatoes, yams, spinach, turnips, all beans and peas.

And we want to make sure to eat the skins of potatoes, yams, and all fruits, with the exception, of course, of melons, bananas, papayas, and pineapples. Whenever we are offered juice, we will ask to eat the entire fruit, with all its fiber. And having committed ourselves to good protein, good fats, and the pursuit of good fiber, the next goal of our diet becomes automatic.

Complex Carbohydrates: High Octane Fuel

Complex carbohydrates, aside from giving us our much-needed fiber, good protein, and rarely any fat, are also our best sources of energy. Unlike refined sugars and carbohydrates, which deliver a jolt of alertness followed by fatigue and depression, foods high in natural sugars metabolize slowly, giving us a steady flow of fuel, keeping us as alert as we can be. Complex carbohydrates contain 100 calories per ounce, but in metabolizing those 100 calories, our body uses 23 calories, and thus they are less easily turned into fat. Recent studies have also found another weight-losing and maintaining function of one particular complex carbohydrate. It seems that jalapeño peppers, if you can tolerate them, can speed up our metabolism, much the way exercise does, causing us to burn calories at a faster rate, turning fewer of them to fat. But that isn't all.

Complex carbohydrates, by which I refer to all fresh vegetables, fruits, and whole grains, supply us with a multitude of vitamins and minerals; they are the best nutrient-per-calorie food around, especially the cruciferous vegetables such as cabbage and broccoli. Without an adequate daily supply of vitamins and minerals, our immune system will be compromised, as will our connective tissue and the hundreds of enzyme systems that run our thinking processes, control inner brain communication, manufacture muscle-cell energy, and are responsible for body movement, coordination, cell replication, regrowth and healing, memory, and total body integrity. Without adequate vitamins and minerals, rejuvenation and longevity are a fantasy.

Looking at it from a positive stance, recent evidence has linked the antioxidant vitamins A, C, and E to neutralization of free radicals and to the prevention of cancerous tumors;

calcium and other minerals are now known to be able to prevent and help treat osteoporosis; the B vitamins and zinc are now closely linked to strong immunity, as are vitamins A, E, and C. And though in the next chapter I will recommend an ambitious vitamin and mineral supplementation plan, there is no question that it is always advantageous to get as many of these elements directly from food as possible. The **Eleventh Goal** of our Rejuvenation Diet, then, is to make complex carbohydrates 60 to 70 percent of our daily caloric intake. When we do so, the next piece of the rejuvenation puzzle should easily fit into place.

Power-Packed Eating: Nutrient Density

Since rejuvenation means limiting calories, it also means getting the maximum number of vitamins, minerals, proteins, carbohydrates, fiber, and essential fatty acids per calorie from our diet. Nutrient density is that ratio, and therefore those foods highest on the nutrient density scale are the best fuel for our bodies. Building a diet around these foods is essential for rejuvenation. Along with the list of foods to follow, I could also document how much of each vitamin and mineral, how much protein, carbohydrate, water-soluble and insoluble fiber, and essential fatty acid it contains and suggest that you start calculating the chemistry of every food in your diet . . . but I won't. It isn't necessary. The **Twelfth Goal** of our Rejuvenation Diet is simply to let these foods become the staple of our diet so that we can get on with the rest of our lives, assured that our eating habits are promoting rejuvenation and longevity.

There have been many studies done on the subject of nutrient density and many lists compiled of the most nutrient-dense foods. Most studies find relatively the same conclusions with only slight variation. My experience in preventive medicine and nutrition and my most recent research leads me to my own set of guidelines in judging the nutrient density of a given food.

> How many of our essential vitamins and minerals can we derive from a single source in relation to its caloric value?

How much water-soluble and water-insoluble fiber does the food contain?

How much protein and how little saturated fat are present?

Is EPA omega-3 essential fatty acid present?

Based on these criteria, my pick for the most nutrient-dense food is parsley. It contains no fat, no cholesterol, and is loaded with vitamins A, C, B-2, B-6; it is a major source of niacin, calcium (more per calorie than milk), magnesium, zinc (more than oysters), potassium (twice as much as a banana), phosphorus, and iron; and it has one calorie per tablespoon. Parsley is full of good fiber and even contains a partial protein.

There is just so much parsley salad, parsley soup, and parsley garnish one can consume, however, so here, in order of nutrient density, are the rest of the most nutrient-dense foods around which we should build our diet:

turnips and turnip greens
bell peppers
collard greens
spinach
carrots
cauliflower
romaine lettuce
Brussels sprouts
asparagus
cantaloupes
papayas, radishes
tomatoes
strawberries
green or yellow squash
cabbage
mushrooms
green beans
cucumbers
oranges
bean sprouts
Shiitake mushrooms
snow peas
celery
grapefruits
fresh or dried apricots
sweet potatoes
green peas
wheat bran
fresh peaches
crab
green onions
watermelons
tuna (fresh or canned in water)
raspberries
eggplant
skim milk
black-eyed peas
sardines (canned in water)
pineapples
wheat germ
lima beans
nonfat yogurt
beets
blueberries
any and all marine fish (such as herring, mackerel, halibut, salmon)
white potatoes
turkey
corn on the cob
cottage cheese
tofu
white meat chicken
cherries
plums
sunflower seeds
bananas
red beans

The list goes on, and there are many other highly nutritious foods to choose from. Nuts, for example, if eaten in small quantities (2 to 3 ounces), are a good source of protein. Any other whole natural food that gives you pleasure should, for that reason, be a part of your Rejuvenation Diet, even if it is not on my list. What we want to do is aim for the foods on this list, knowing they are the best fuel on which we can run our bodies. And we don't have to calculate. If we eat fruits, vegetables, beans, and grains in their natural whole state (not as refined flour or juice) our bodies will get the fiber we need without our ever having to make a conscious effort toward a high-fiber diet. If we eat a wide variety of nutrient-dense foods we will, without having to measure, calculate, or analyze, be eating a truly well-balanced diet, as well as strengthening our immune system and promoting longevity.

We also do not need to concern ourselves with specific food combinations. In recent years, there has been a lot of talk about food combining—don't eat protein with starch and don't eat fruit with anything—and I have yet to be convinced that there is any validity whatsoever to these claims. My greatest objection to these theories is their assumption that a piece of chicken is protein and nothing more, and a potato is a complex carbohydrate only. This, as you and I already know, is not true. It is impossible to eat carbohydrate without combining it with protein since every carbohydrate contains at least some protein. What convinces me most relating to any theory of nutrition are studies of societies in which many people live into their second century—and none of these people knows anything about food combining. If we are really concerned about getting iron from our diet, it is true that we can boost iron intake by combining high-iron foods with high–vitamin C foods—for a example lima beans with red peppers or figs with cantaloupe—but basically we are *what* we eat, not what we eat it with.

What we eat, however, does depend to a large degree on how we cook it and how well we chew it.

STEAMING YOUR WAY TO GOOD HEALTH: FOOD PREPARATION

A potato is one of the best pure foods nature has to offer us. It contains a measurable amount of protein, lots of potassium, iron, calcium, niacin, vitamins A, B-2, and C, complex carbohydrates, and good fiber, with 90 to 110 calories and almost no fat per the average potato. French fried potatoes, however, usually deep-fried in animal lard, are one of the most unhealthy foods, being high in saturated fat, with two to three times as many calories and almost none of the nutrients left; and potato chips are completely void of nutrients, being almost pure fat and containing four to five times as many calories as the original potato from which they were made. Even boiling a potato, while it does not add fat or calories, does drain the potato of much of its nutrient value, which ends up in the boiled water and steam.

How a food is prepared can have as much of an effect on our health as what the food was to begin with. So the **Thirteenth Goal** of our Rejuvenation Diet is to prepare our food in the most nutritious (and delicious) way possible. This, of course, is different for different kinds of rejuvenation foods.

Our fish, skinless poultry, flank steak, or lean leg of lamb should be either steamed, or baked *below* the flame, without butter or any kind of oil. Any time a fat drips onto a flame it is turned into a mutagen, making our food carcinogenic. In fact, it was recently discovered that an average piece of barbecued or broiled meat contains more carcinogens than 600 cigarettes. Furthermore, no meat or fish should ever be eaten raw, including clams, oysters, and, yes—sushi. While raw fish may be fashionable, it can cause a number of gastrointestinal diseases (which are not so fashionable), as well as cholera, hepatitis, vibrio, paralytic shellfish poisoning, and a number of bacterial and viral infections. Steaming clams and oysters is only truly safe if done for *at least six minutes.* Otherwise they can be contaminated with any number of pathogens.

Vegetables are often best raw, especially carrots, peppers,

and leafy greens. Lightly steaming may enhance flavor without removing too many nutrients or too much fiber. As a general rule, with most foods the longer you cook, the less valuable the food becomes to your body. The longer you let a food stew, brew, or bake, the more you are oxidizing, diluting, and dripping out all the nutrients. We cannot get nourishment by breathing vitamins and minerals through kitchen aromas. Potatoes and yams must, of course, be sufficiently cooked; baking or sufficient microwaving I find the best way. Popcorn should be done in an air popper, which needs no oil, and beans are best boiled, baked, or microwaved.

Sometimes the best kind of cooking is no cooking at all, as with fruits—though an occasional baked apple is a fine treat—and especially with bread. Toasting bread, even those of the good, honest whole-grain variety, it has recently been found, destroys most of its protein, changing the amino acids to nonusable types. The more brown you make bread the less nutritious even the best slice will become. Warming bread in an oven or microwave, however, is fine.

And regardless of what Rejuvenation Diet food choices we make or how we choose to safely prepare them, the **Fourteenth Goal** of our Rejuvenation Diet is to chew our food at least fifty times before swallowing. This gives our saliva a chance to really mix with the food and begin digestion. Swallowing food that has not been sufficiently chewed causes inadequate breakdown of the cellular content of the food so that the nutritive value contained within those food cells may likely pass through us and be excreted without fueling us at all.

Eating the foods recommended in this diet will make adequate chewing much easier, since we are eating foods in their whole, natural state. Crunchy vegetables, pasta, and brown rice require extensive chewing, unlike white bread and other junk food which slide down the throat before our teeth can get any hold on them.

Finally, the best reason of all to chew food thoroughly is that it is an effective cure for overeating and obesity. Adequate chewing gives the stomach that twenty minutes it needs to tell the brain it is full. Chewing thoroughly gives our mouths a chance to taste the food, giving us a chance to enjoy all the sensory experiences of eating: the smell, sight, taste, touch, even the sound. Eating fast—whether it is fast food or not—is cheating yourself out of one of the most universally enjoyable human experiences.

ENJOY YOURSELF

Following the Rejuvenation Diet may sometimes be painstaking, but it should never be painful. The **Fifteenth Goal** of our Rejuvenation Diet is to make our daily diet as pleasurable as possible. This means variety, seasoning; it means becoming a gourmet without the sugar, the salt, or the cream. I do not believe in handing out specific menus to my patients or to anyone; but just as an example, let me share with you some typical meals I try to treat myself to:

GREAT BREAKFASTS

1. Half grapefruit or papaya or banana or one orange; ⅔ cup of cereal (hot: oatmeal, cream of wheat, kasha or kashi, seven grain, millet; cold: kashi, shredded wheat, Nutri-grain corn or wheat and raisins, puffed wheat, rice, or corn); add 1 tsp wheat germ plus ½ cup of nonfat milk; plus any caffeine substitute breakfast drink such as commercial herb tea.
2. Two-thirds cup of nonfat yogurt mixed with sliced banana, ½ orange, 1 tsp raisins, 1 tsp wheat germ; two slices whole wheat, sour dough, or rye bread; plus noncaffeine beverage.
3. One large baked yam (hot or cold); one glass nonfat milk; two hardboiled egg *whites.*

GREAT LUNCHES

1. Salad of mixed greens and other raw vegetables; one 3.5 oz can of water-packed tuna or 3 oz of unprocessed white breast of turkey with onions, garlic, and olive oil.
2. Pasta (preferably fresh and whole grain) in a water-base tomato sauce with oregano and peppers.

3. Japanese sushi (nonraw type).
4. Two oz nonfat (or 1% lowfat) cottage cheese and a large multi-fruit salad.

GREAT DINNERS

1. Small dinner salad with a variety of fresh raw vegetables (carrots, cauliflower, etc.) and a yogurt dip; up to 6 oz of fresh deep-water fish, poached, broiled (under flame), or baked; two green vegetables and one yellow vegetable, steamed.
2. Large, raw, multi vegetable salad with 1 oz grated mozzarella cheese, dressed with 1 tbls olive oil, apple cider vinegar, and fresh (not powdered) garlic.
3. Salad of raw vegetables; white meat turkey; yams or sweet potatoes.
4. Beans with rice or kasha; 1 oz cheddar cheese.
5. Pasta noodles, hot, with ½ cup nonfat or 1% lowfat cottage cheese.
6. One steamed lobster, asparagus and carrots, one medium baked potato, one green vegetable, fresh fruit.

GREAT SNACKS

1. Up to 1 quart of dry, air-popped popcorn.
2. Fresh or dried fruit; frozen banana.
3. One to three large raw carrots.
4. Cold cooked slices yam, sweetened with one to four drops of blackstrap molasses, refrigerated or frozen.

Eating in restaurants should not be an obstacle to growing younger. Fish and chicken are on most all menus, as are salads and other fresh vegetables. The last time I ate out, this is what I ordered: hearts of lettuce with tomato juice as dressing, poached salmon, steamed broccoli and asparagus (hold the hollandaise sauce, please), baked potato (no butter, no salt, no sour cream), and a piece of melon for desert. As people become more aware of good nutrition, most good restaurants try to be accommodating to the customer who is trying to stay healthy. Many lunch menus are now dominated by salads, and many breakfast places now offer whole-grain cereals and a variety of fresh fruits.

Do not expect yourself to change the minute you close this book. If you do make a 360° turn, that's terrific; but if not, don't give up. What we need above all else is the *desire* to change; the desire to grow younger and live longer better. Every year in this country a staggering 125,000 people die because they neglected to take their heart medicine; they obviously did not care a heck of a lot about their health. If you really care about your good health then you're a lot better off than a lot of people. But don't stop here. The **Final Goal** of our Rejuvenation Diet is to complement it with supplemental insurance: a careful look at medicines, a rigorous program of daily exercise, and a healthy mental outlook. Diet is only one piece of the rejuvenation puzzle.

3 Vitamin and Mineral Insurance

There is a substantial group of reputable medical thinkers today who deny that nutritional supplements have any role in rejuvenation or longevity. They make a persuasive argument, an argument that seems logical and hard to disagree with. They point to fraudulent claims made by vitamin enthusiasts of miracle cures using megadoses, and they are absolutely correct in that assertion; there are a lot of unqualified people recommending vitamins, minerals, and amino acids they know little or nothing about. The anti-supplement doctors go on to suggest that all we really need is to eat a well-balanced diet along the lines of the Rejuvenation Diet, and they maintain that if we do so we will consume all of our essential vitamins and minerals and have no need for supplements. This is, as I will soon explain, wishful thinking. Other doctors do personally recognize the necessity of supplementing a healthy diet with vitamins, minerals, and certain amino acids, but they are afraid to start recommending them to their patients because it might go against the current consensus of the medical community. I once caught a colleague of mine, who publicly dismisses supplements, in a vitamin store loading up on his own personal supply. It is slightly absurd that a doctor should think he is going out on a limb to recommend a few thousand milligrams of vitamin C in a world where cattle ranchers inject hormones into their livestock, municipalities dump chlorine (a known carcinogen) into their water supplies, while produce companies irradiate much of our "fresh" produce. Nevertheless, here I am out on a limb advising you, based on my twenty-three years of practicing preventive medicine, to complement a healthy intake of food with a healthy intake of vitamin, mineral, and perhaps the occasional amino acid or essential fatty acid supplement.

There are an array of convincing reasons. If, as I have suggested, we maintain a low caloric intake, it is next to impossible for us to get enough of every single vitamin, mineral, and amino acid our bodies need. Take iron for example. The average woman needs 18 milligrams per day; a diet high in iron-packed foods, however, only gives her about 6 milligrams per 1000 calories. This means she must consume 3000 calories per day, as much as twice the healthful amount, in order to get her daily iron requirements from her "well-balanced" diet (and this assumes that her body will absorb all it needs and that other iron-blocking foods are not present to sabotage absorption).

Then there is the problem of complexity. No doctor is going to sit down with you and calculate the nutrients in each food in your diet and formulate a plan to cover your every nutrient need. (The only professionals who do this are zoo keepers whose job it is to keep their animals healthy, as opposed to treating them once they are sick.) If we tried to calculate the perfect and complete diet ourselves, it would take about three hours a day, which I don't think is anyone's idea of a good time. And even so, we could still never be sure.

Each of us maintains his or her own biochemical individuality, so that nutritional needs vary from person to person and change under a variety of conditions such as age, size, illness, and stress. Furthermore, not everyone absorbs all the vitamins and minerals from their diet—some people do not absorb nearly enough—so this idea of an "average" requirement of a "normal" person is absurd. Each of us is a unique organism with our own biochemical individuality. Many of us need far more than than what the FDA or the USDA or the National Academy of Scientists say we need. Moreover, we must consider the assault that much of our food must endure: the spraying, the possibility that the "fresh produce" we are eating has been stored in a silo for three years and dyed back to life, the misguided packaging of foods (so that, for example, the riboflavin in milk in a see-through plastic container disintegrates when exposed to light), and the great variety of chemical changes that happen to food during storage, transportation, and whatever we might do to it while cooking (or burning). So you can see why the insurance of supplements makes a lot of sense. If you are still not convinced, consider the fact that there are other essential nutrients that exist in large supply only in foods that are otherwise unhealthy. If we eliminate red meat completely from our diet, or eat it very seldom, then we are probably going to be deficient in iron and in L-carnitine, an important amino acid. And finally, some people's daily needs of certain minerals—for example, calcium, which is crucial to preventing osteoporosis—are so high that they could not hope to meet them even if they consumed hundreds of extra calories of dairy products per day.

In no way do I mean to suggest that supplements are any kind of substitute for good nutrition. We cannot expect to strengthen our immune system and grow younger by eating processed junk and chasing it down with some vitamin, mineral, and amino acid pills. There is also no denying that too much of any supplement can be unhealthy, although nothing I suggest is anywhere near a toxic level. There is nothing magic implied in a supplementation program. It is only a small piece of the longevity puzzle, but an important one, and certainly an easy piece to provide.

Our goal with supplements is to consume safe but effective amounts of all the vitamins and minerals, and possibly some extra amino acids, needed for continuing rejuvenation, and to do so in the simplest possible manner. There are quite a few good books on vitamins, which I will recommend in the back of this book, but you don't have to read them. While it is a good idea to seek individual guidance from your own physician to see if you have any allergies to any vitamins or minerals, all you probably need to know, and all you need to take, follows in these next pages. For most of my patients over the years this has meant finding the best possible multivitamin and multimineral supplement, to which they add single tablets of those vitamins, minerals, amino acids and/or essential fatty acids of which their bodies require large amounts. First, I will share my knowledge and medical experience of these requirements, then briefly discuss the best, least intrusive approach to meeting them.

TAKE YOUR VITAMINS: THE SIX ESSENTIALS

Vitamin A is essential to the maintenance of a strong immune system; it enhances the production of macrophage defender cells, as well as our T-cells responsible for stimulating interleukin. Vitamin A inhibits inflammations such as arthritis, myositis, and tendonitis, and can be helpful in fighting such skin diseases as eczema, acne, and psoriasis. It is no secret that vitamin A is vital to good eyesight (though this is true only if our bodies have an adequate supply of the mineral *zinc*); but vitamin A is also now known to slow the aging of cellular material and to possibly prevent cancer by enhancing our white blood cells. Vitamin A deficiency can cause dry eyes, eye inflammation, inflamed eyelids, corneal ulcers, night blindness, dry skin, brittle nails, poor hair quality, fatigue, diarrhea, reduced sense of smell and taste, and consequently poor appetite; also poor bones and teeth, poor wound healing, reduced integrity of all cells lining our insides, and reduced immunity. A lack of vitamin A also greatly diminishes our body's ability to use vitamin C.

If any of these symptoms sound familiar, you may soon be able to bid them farewell. There are many good natural food sources of vitamin A—especially dark green and orange vegetables—but to ensure an adequate daily supply of this essential vitamin, I recommend 10,000 to 25,000 units daily. Since excessive doses of this vitamin can be toxic, causing liver disease, headaches, hair loss (and can even in some cases be fatal) you will want to take it in the safer form of its precursor, *beta carotene,* which is now used in many good multivitamin tablets. Your body's immediate vitamin A needs will determine how much of the beta carotene it will convert to vitamin A, thus likely eliminating any possibility of toxicity. (If you have had any history of liver disorders, I urge you to have your physician check your ability to metabolize and tolerate beta carotene).

The B vitamins, thiamin (B-1), riboflavin (B-2), niacin (B-3), pantothenic acid (B-5), pyridoxine (B-6), cobalamin (B-12), biotin, choline, inositol, para-aminobenzoic acid (PABA), and folic acid are important in our energy production and the burning up of carbohydrates as fuel. They help maintain the integrity and function of the nervous system, the muscles, the skin, as well as the metabolic functions in the liver, the enzymes which process all chemical reactions of our food, fuels, hormones, and detoxification. Some of the more recent and exciting discoveries about the B vitamins are that niacin appears to lower cholesterol and reduce the chance of heart disease; pantothenic acid appears to help prevent, or at least lessen the symptoms of, rheumatoid arthritis and other autoimmune diseases in some people; B-6 has been found to neutralize free radicals which cause tumors and, for many people, has been known to reduce the occurrence of asthma; and all the B-vitamins are now known to be crucial in the fortification of our immune system.

There are many good food sources of the B-vitamins: most whole grains, nonfat dairy, most beans, many vegetables, especially leafy greens. There are also many unpleasant symptoms of vitamin B deficiency—poor digestion, weak heart muscle, fatigue, irritability and nervousness, tender muscles, and liver disease—all good reasons to seek the nutritional insurance of a B-complex supplement. There is a delicate balance between the various B vitamins—too much of one can wipe out the others—so they must be taken together and each must be taken in sufficient amounts to support any extra dosage of any single B vitamin, such as niacin. The daily dosages to look for in a multivitamin or a B-complex tablet are:

Thiamin (B-1)	15 to 100 mgs*
Riboflavin (B-2)	30 to 50 mgs
Niacin (B-3)	30 to 50 mgs**
Pantothenic acid (B-5)	50 to 250 mgs*
Pyridoxine (B-6)	25 to 50 mgs
Cobalamin (B-12)	100 to 400 micrograms (mcgs)
Biotin	50 mgs
Choline	1000 mgs
Inositol	100 mgs
PABA	40 mgs
Folic acid	400 micrograms (mcgs)*

Vitamin C (ascorbic acid) plays a major role in sustaining our immunity at an optimum level; it helps protect our body against oxidizing chemicals and free radicals which are now known to destroy cells and cause tumors. Ascorbic acid helps to block the formation of blood clots and thus protects against heart attack and stroke. Experimental studies suggest that vitamin C may offer some protection against certain cancers, in-

*Our need for thiamin/B-1, pantothenic acid, and folic acid can become two to ten times as great if we are ill, under stress, or on certain medications—in which case we may require an extra B-1, B-5, and folic acid supplement.

**If you take niacin in the form of niacinamide you will need 100 milligrams.

cluding cancer of the bladder and large intestine. In fact, renowned scientist Linus Pauling believes that megadoses of vitamin C can greatly reduce our risk of all types of cancers. His theories have yet to win acceptance among the medical establishment. Yet since we know that 10,000 to 20,000 milligrams of vitamin C is usually not dangerous unless there is already a condition of kidney disease or gout, many health-conscious people, including myself and many of my patients, have gone ahead and taken megadoses of ascorbic acid in the hope that Pauling's conclusion will prove true, like so many scientific realities that take years to become "officially" recognized. Already, some of the most conservative medical journals have published findings linking vitamin C deficiency with cancer and heart disease, and connecting high levels of vitamin C with increased levels of HDL "good guy" cholesterol.

With that in mind, you may want to try 6000 to 10,000 milligrams a day or to tolerance, keeping an awareness of the potential side effects: nausea, diarrhea, abdominal cramps. If any of these begin to occur, you may want to cut down to a more moderate dosage. My *minimum* daily dosage of vitamin C, however, is much higher than the RDA's recommendation of 60 milligrams. Experience tells me that we need at least 1000 to 2000 milligrams to help us grow—and stay—younger. Few multivitamins contain this much ascorbic acid, and while there are a lot of good and well-known food sources of vitamin C, like citrus fruits and dark green vegetables, it is difficult to ingest 1000 milligrams every single day, so you will likely need to take a separate vitamin C supplement in addition to your multivitamin. Since vitamin C boosts the absorption of iron and of calcium, always take at least some of your vitamin C along with your calcium; and if you are taking an iron supplement you should chase it down with some of your vitamin C. Since vitamin C is destroyed by alcohol, barbiturates, antibiotics, aspirin, hormone drugs, tobacco, and baking soda, the amount of benefit you are likely to derive from ascorbic acid may depend on your intake, or avoidance, of these substances.

An interesting warning has recently arisen regarding the

effects of vitamin C on those fish containing mercury. Problem: it seems that vitamin C, if taken with such fish, releases toxic mercury that would otherwise not be available for metabolism. Answer: if you have any reason to suspect that there is mercury in the fish you are eating, do not take your vitamin C with it.

Vitamin D is needed to regulate and metabolize calcium, and thus is vital for strong bones and the prevention of osteoporosis. Vitamin D is also needed in fortifying our nervous system and skin. Dairy products, egg yolks, organ meats, and direct sunlight possess the highest content of vitamin D; and since we want to drastically reduce our intake of most of these things, including sunlight which over time can cause skin cancer, our rejuvenation plan calls for 400 International Units (IUs) of vitamin D per day. This amount is added to most commercially sold quarts of nonfat milk and may be obtained by drinking a quart of milk daily. Otherwise, 400 IUs of vitamin D should be easy to find in a good multivitamin capsule.

Vitamin E can improve our memory and enhance our immune system. It is vital to the maintenance of all tissue and is needed for healthy blood circulation. As an antioxident, it is now known to help neutralize free radicals which are now believed responsible for deterioration and disease once thought to be the result of aging. In recent studies, vitamin E has been shown to reduce the incidence of tumors, lower cholesterol, and neutralize toxic substances in the body to slow aging. Good food sources of vitamin E are wheat germ, soybeans, dark green vegetables, brown rice, nuts, and many fruits. I generally prescribe 100 to 400 IUs daily to make sure my patients get enough of it. This amount can often be found in a good multivitamin tablet. I have prescribed as much as 800 IUs daily, especially for patients with high cholesterol, but always with the following warnings: vitamin E can cause fatigue and gastrointestinal problems; it may, in high doses, cause easy bleeding and should not be taken with aspirin or any anticoagulent medication; it can cause blood clots or elevate blood pressure. Any of these adverse effects obviously indicate the need to decrease dosage back to between 100 and 400 IUs.

Vitamin K is the last of the essential vitamins. Without it, our blood will not clot properly. But this key vitamin is so plentiful in any healthy diet (and much of it is produced in our own colon and intestinal tract) that I advise my patients to stay away from supplements containing vitamin K—especially if they are on blood-thinning heart medicines.

What we are looking for, then, is a multivitamin that contains the right amounts of vitamin A (as *beta carotene*), the B vitamins, vitamin D, and vitamin E. Add to that a daily vitamin C dosage of at least 1000 milligrams and, depending on how elaborate we want our rejuvenation insurance to be, perhaps some additional niacin, vitamin E, and beta carotene. The label of our multivitamin should look something like this:

Beta carotene	10,000 to 25,000 IUs
Thiamin (B-1)	15 to 100 mgs
Riboflavin (B-2)	30 to 50 mgs
Niacin (B-3)	30 to 50 mgs
Pantothenic acid (B-5)	50 to 250 mgs
Pyridoxine (B-6)	25 to 50 mgs
Cobalamin (B-12)	100 to 400 mcgs
Biotin	50 mgs
Choline	1000 mgs
Inositol	100 mgs
PABA	40 mgs
Folic acid	400 mcgs
Vitamin D	400 IUs
Vitamin E	100 to 400 IUs

In addition, we want in a separate tablet:

Vitamin C	1000 to 2000 mgs

Even if we decide to try more than 2000 milligrams per day, it is best to space it out over the course of the day.

THE CASE FOR MINERAL SUPPLEMENTS

Like the B vitamins, minerals can only work in our bodies to aid in the rejuvenation process if taken in combination with one another. There are two types of minerals: macrominerals, of which we need calcium, iron, magnesium, and phosphorus, and trace minerals, of which we need copper, chromium, manganese, selenium, and zinc. New theories exist suggesting we also may need cobalt, molybdenum, vanadium, silicon, and rubidium in such infinitesimal amounts that only in rare cases would we not get enough of them from our diet. Trace minerals are toxic in large doses. This is why we recommend milligrams of the macrominerals and *micrograms* of the trace minerals. There are a lot of good multimineral supplements that contain most of the important minerals at good insurance dosages, but certain key minerals are needed in such great quantities that they must be swallowed separately.

One such crucial mineral is *calcium.* It is essential to strong bones and teeth and the prevention of osteoporosis; it is crucial for normal blood clotting, and to our nervous system, heart rhythm, muscle function, and cellular metabolism. There are many good dietary sources for calcium—skim milk and lowfat yogurt, green vegetables, root vegetables, sardines and salmon, and tofu—but as our years increase, our need for this mineral increases so much that it can be impossible to get our daily requirement from our diet. I recommend at least 1500 milligrams daily of supplemental calcium. Since for yet uncertain reasons calcium seems to be better absorbed later in the day, I have my patients take half with lunch and half with dinner; and I make certain to remind them to keep a ratio of 2:1 calcium to magnesium. If this ratio is not maintained, any large doses of calcium can block absorption of magnesium. Another potential risk of large amounts of calcium may be the development of kidney stones, though there is not yet enough supportive evidence of that fact to give it much consideration with respect to the importance of an adequate daily intake of calcium. Vitamin C helps in the absorption of calcium, as do unsaturated fatty acids found in fish and soybeans. Aspirin antagonizes calcium in the body, and the two should not be taken at the same time.

There are many forms of calcium supplements. The most convenient is calcium carbonate, which can be safely taken up to my recommended dosage. Some antacid companies have recently been boasting that their heartburn remedy contains calcium, but I hardly think antacid is the wisest means to fill your daily requirement. What these drug companies do not tell you is that the amount of calcium is far lower than is needed for any realistic rejuvenation plan, and also that the aluminum content of their product is much higher than our bodies can afford. Moreover, they fail to mention that calcium needs stomach acid (which antacid depletes) to be properly absorbed, that calcium will not work at all unless it is complemented by an adequate supply of zinc, and that calcium is not the only mineral needed for durable bones.

Copper is just as important, not only to bone formation but to red blood cell integrity, skin and immune functions, nervous system functions, the conversion of beta carotene to vitamin A, and the processing of vitamin C. Without an adequate supply of copper, skin becomes fragile, will break easily, and heal slowly, bones will fracture easily, blood vessels can leak or even burst and cause an aneurysm. There are many healthy foods rich in copper, such as whole grains, leafy greens, almonds, most fish, most beans, avocados, cauliflower, raisins, and steamed oysters, but no one should risk a deficiency of this key element, so we want our multimineral tablets to contain 2 milligrams of copper, best taken along with zinc; and we want to remember that excess refined sugar can wipe out our copper supply.

Chromium, another important mineral, is vital to our ability to provide insulin, metabolize carbohydrates into energy, metabolize fatty acids and cholesterol, stabilize blood sugar, and synthesize protein. It can be eaten in brewer's yeast, nonfat dairy products, whole grains, black pepper, and mushrooms. But to ensure that we are getting enough, our multimineral supplement should contain about 100 to 150 micrograms of this element.

Iron is another essential mineral, needed for healthy red and white blood cells, efficient oxygen use and energy production, muscle and thyroid functions, immune system integrity, protein metabolism, and a variety of cognitive brain functions. It is no secret that iron deficiency causes fatigue and irritability, but recent evidence also suggests that a lack of iron in our blood can lower our resistance to recurring infections. We've learned that an iron deficiency may exist without anemia, so if you are experiencing some of these symptoms but your doctor tells you you're not anemic and assumes therefore that you're not iron deficient, have him do a serum iron level check, called a *ferritin.*

It is well known that spinach is a good source of iron, but so are other leafy greens, as well as fish, steamed oysters, wheat germ, legumes, poultry, and whole grains. Women tend to need about 33 percent more iron than men, and if we are taking adequate levels of calcium we will increase our need for iron. Because of complications connected with taking excess iron, such as gas, diarrhea, suppressed immunity, free radical enhancement, vitamin E destruction, and liver problems, I cannot recommend that everyone take it in a supplemental form. For my own patients, when I discover an iron deficiency, through taking a serum ferritin check, I usually prescribe a chelated iron tablet of 99 milligrams (or, if needed, a more potent form of ferrous gluconate) along with an extra 1000 to 2000 milligrams of vitamin C. I am among those in the medical profession who believes that iron in a chelated form, meaning that it is attached to a protein molecule, is more easily absorbed, creating less gastric upset, and therefore the best supplemental form, especially for the person with an iron absorption problem. Other doctors, however, may not feel this way; and since an iron deficiency is a medical problem requiring the treatment of a physician, I cannot outright recommend chelated iron over the ferrous gluconate. I can, however, remind you to take any prescribed iron supplement with vitamin C, and separate from all other minerals.

Another key mineral, one often overlooked, is *magnesium,* which is necessary for the maintaining of healthy bones, normal heart rhythm, the proper function of nerves and muscles, maintenance of PH balance of blood and tissue, and metabolism of carbohydrates, calcium, vitamin D, amino acids, and essential fatty acids. The most recent studies now indicate magnesium's important role in strengthening the immune system and lowering cholesterol. One recent study found that people suffering coronaries had very low levels of magnesium in their bodies; and while scientists have not yet determined if the coronary caused the deficiency or the deficiency was part of the cause of the coronary, the finding still underscores the importance of this mineral. Magnesium deficiency may be the most common and most overlooked mineral deficiency in America today, especially with the new emphasis on calcium, which uses magnesium in its own absorption and can, if we do not compensate for this, leave the body deficient in this essential element. A deficiency can cause irritability, anxiety, and night cramps, especially in the legs; it can expedite the onset of osteoporosis or worsen an already existing instance.

Good dietary sources of magnesium include whole grains, shellfish, seafood, dark greens, soybean products, bananas, cashews, almonds, and most seeds. Foods that can rob magnesium from us are saturated fats and, in particular, soda pop, which is high in phosphates. The RDA is 300 milligrams of magnesium for women, 350 for men. My own reading and medical experience, however, lead me to suggest double those amounts—600 milligrams for women, 700 for men—especially if you are now experiencing any of the deficiency symptoms. It is unlikely you will find this much in a multimineral, so you will have to look for it as a separate supplement. Make sure not to take more than 1000 mgs; too much magnesium can cause kidney trouble and heart rhythm irregularities. Anyone with heart block should consult his or her physician before taking any magnesium supplement.

Manganese is yet another element crucial to the prevention of osteoporosis. It is also essential for the metabolizing of the B vitamins, vitamin C, carbohydrates, fats, and proteins.

We cannot maintain healthy bones without an adequate supply of this mineral. Nor can we be sure our nervous system and blood formation are as viable as possible without manganese. Whole grains, green vegetables, celery, bananas, pineapples, and most beans are good dietary sources. Recent studies, however, show that many people do not properly absorb manganese from the foods they eat; and since there are no known cases of nutrient manganese toxicity with levels up to 15 milligrams, a good supplemental program should include 10 to 15 milligrams of this essential element. Until a few years ago it was somewhat rare to find manganese in a multimineral tablet, but the growing awareness of how important this mineral is has begun to make it available in this form. I suspect that within a few years no good multimineral will be without it.

We need *potassium* to regulate the balance of sodium and water in our body, and to maintain a healthy nervous system, muscle function, amino acid metabolism, and heart rhythm. Major sources of potassium include almost all vegetables and many fruits (especially oranges and bananas), as well as whole grains, sunflower seeds, potatoes (especially the skin), dates, figs, apricots, lima beans, and seafood. In fact, potassium is so easily available in a healthy rejuvenation diet that it is *not* imperative, or even advisable, to take it at all in supplemental form. Excess potassium can endanger heart rhythms. This is why excess salt substitutes, which are full of potassium, are dangerous.

Another key mineral is *selenium*, needed to fight cell damage from free radicals and oxidation, and important in the development of antibodies, protection against heart disease, and general immunity. The latest study on selenium content in soil throughout the world revealed an interesting finding: those parts of the world with high selenium content in their soil had a much lower cancer rate than parts of the world where soil was low in selenium. Whole grains, wheat germ, broccoli, onions, tomatoes, and tuna are good bets for selenium in the diet, and a good daily insurance of selenium can range from 100 to 150 micrograms, *no more.* Too much of this mineral can be toxic. You may be able to find the right amount of selenium in a multimineral, but you will most likely have to get it in a separate tablet. For some people, even the usual safe dosage can cause blackening of fingernails or nausea; if these side effects occur, stop supplemental selenium at once.

Finally, we come to *zinc.* This trace mineral has become a focal point in both nutritional and medical circles, primarily because of its key role in achieving a healthy immune system. If our body does not maintain a sufficient level of zinc, our protector T-cells will not form and our white blood cell count may become very low, leaving us vulnerable to any number of viral and bacterial infections. Zinc deficiency, in fact, is common among people most susceptible to colds and flu, and can also impair your sense of taste and smell, severely impede the healing process, and *may* be a factor contributing to male impotency. The body does not store zinc, and thus it must be taken every day to ensure good health and continuing rejuvenation. Good food sources of zinc are oysters (never eaten raw, please), sprouts, dark greens, sauerkraut, pumpkin, squash, onions, and sesame and sunflower seeds. But, so that you don't have to keep tabs on your zinc intake, I suggest a supplement containing 10 to 15 milligrams daily; a good multimineral tablet should contain this much. Since zinc interacts with copper, it must be balanced in a ratio of from 7:1 to 10:1 zinc to copper. If zinc is allowed to block copper absorption, it can raise serum cholesterol. Too much zinc can also interact with iron to cause an anemia. If you follow my recommendations, however, and find a good multimineral supplement, you will not have to worry or calculate.

There are other minerals we need, such as salt, iodine, and phosphorus, but most of us are already getting too much of these, so we want to make sure our mineral supplement *does not* contain them. The ideal multimineral tablet contains my recommended amounts of copper, manganese, selenium, and zinc. You will probably need separate tablets of calcium, magnesium, and iron if you are diagnosed with a deficiency. If, however, it is difficult for you to find a multimineral containing enough manganese or selenium (the importance of these has just lately been documented), you may want to go for separate tablets of them as well, though I predict that as the evidence of their importance mounts, it will be hard to find a good multimineral that is short on manganese or selenium. The label of our multimineral, then, should probably look something like this:

Copper	2 mgs
Chromium	100 to 150 mcgs
Manganese	10 to 15 mgs
Zinc	15 mgs

In addition, if we cannot find these in our multimineral, we may need separate tablets of:

Magnesium	500 to 750 mgs
Manganese	10 to 15 mgs
Selenium	100 to 150 mcgms

And we will definitely want separate tablets of:

Calcium	1500 mgs
Iron	as per doctor, if deficiency is found

THE PROTEIN CONNECTION: AMINO ACID SUPPLEMENTS

Some of the newest and most exciting nutritional discoveries of the last few years, and in my opinion the new frontier of nutrition and preventive medicine, involve the amino acids. There are many of these complex building blocks in proteins, and they interact with one another in numerous ways. So far, there are five that have received attention from medical researchers and seem to be important enough to warrant the attention of anyone interested in good health and longevity. Since there is much yet to be learned about them, I cannot recommend them unreservedly. They are a double-edged sword, with benefits as well as potential side effects; but I can bring them to your attention. If you decide that you do want to try them, start out at the low end of the dosage, and if desired results occur, slowly increase your daily supplemental intake. A sudden high dosage might have undesirable results.

L-arginine is essential to our immune system, growth hormones, tissue repair and formation, and fat metabolism. It seems to stimulate healing and may play a role in cancer prevention. If you eat a lot of nuts, seeds, and beans, it is likely you are getting enough—and it is always preferable to get it from food. If not, a supplement of 500 to 600 milligrams might be in order. Potential side effects are that it can support an existing herpes virus, causing the onset of lesions.

There are now reports that the amino acid *L-cystine* may relieve arthritis and may in general be able to extend our lifespan. Though further study is needed in these areas, the word in thus far on cystine is exciting. It appears to aid in the repair and maintenance of our central intelligence system, and among other possible uses it may be protective against certain carcinogens. Thus far the known side effects of supplemental cystine are that it can antagonize insulin in diabetics and may increase the headaches produced by monosodium glutamate. Excess cystine may also form kidney stones (though this can be prevented easily by consuming vitamin C at a ratio of 2:1 over cystine supplement). The best food sources of cystine are nonfat yogurt and whole grains. If you decide to take it as a supplement, I recommend not taking more than 500 milligrams.

L-tryptophan represents one of the most exciting recent medical discoveries. It is now known to be vital to the brain process of converting *serotonin*, a chemical messenger in the brain that is essential for relaxation and good sleep. It may prove to be beneficial in dealing with insomnia as well as stress, depression, and chronic pain. It has, in fact, been used in fairly high dosages as a sleeping aid, but there may be side effects. Some limited studies involving laboratory animals linked such high doses of L-tryptophan to liver disease and to bladder cancer in those lab animals purposefully deficient in vitamin B-6. Thus far, however, there are no conclusive studies pointing to any side effects using reasonable doses of this amino acid. Nonfat milk is a good source, as are bananas and turkey. A safe and effective supplemental dosage should be somewhere between 500 and 2000 milligrams.

Lysine is involved with tissue repair and formation, and can also suppress the herpes virus. Lowfat milk products, fish, fowl, and brewer's yeast are good food sources, and 500 to 3000 milligrams in supplemental form is part of good rejuvenation insurance. For my patients with active herpes I prescribe 500 milligrams four times daily. There are no *known* side effects.

L-carnitine is needed in our bodies for energy production, to regulate fat metabolism, and to regulate the metabolism and contractive strength of the heart and skeletal muscles. It is bound to become a recognized part of cardiac therapy and may very well prove to be helpful in dealing with muscular dystrophy and other muscle disorders. L-carnitine is substantially present only in red meat. This means that if, as I strongly suggest, you eliminate or drastically cut down on your consumption of red meat (and certainly if you are a vegetarian), it is more than likely that you are going to be deficient in L-carnitine. L-carnitine deficiency can cause muscle fatigue, cramps, and—after exercise—a condition called myoglobulinuria, in which certain muscles break down and are excreted in the urine. I have prescribed L-carnitine supplements to any patient complaining of fatigue (especially those who are eating well and exercising regularly), and have seen tremendous results. There are no known side effects, which has led the FDA to recently approve its use. I suggest a daily dosage of 500 to 3000 milligrams—and make sure you take *L-carnitine* not *DL-carnitine,* which is potentially toxic.

Another important amino acid, *DL-phenylalanine,* prolongs the life of our body's endorphins and enkephalins (both mood elevating, depression-fighting chemicals produced inside us primarily from exercise). It is present primarily in animal protein, and if you drastically cut down your consumption of animal protein, as I recommend, you may want to add 100 to 3000 milligrams of this amino acid to your supplementation program.

FISH OIL AND CHARCOAL

You may also want to consider supplementing omega-3, EPA fish oil tablets. While they are no substitute for a diet featuring deep-water fish, they may be good insurance (especially for vegetarians) against high cholesterol, high blood pressure, heart disease, rheumatoid arthritis, and perhaps even cancer. 120 to 1800 milligrams is probably the safe and effective daily supplemental dosage range; but bear in mind that no dosage has actually been established, that EPA capsules cause diarrhea in some people, that they *may* reduce blood clotting to the point of causing excessive bleeding from a cut or spontaneous bleeding, and that aspirin and/or anti-blood clot therapy should probably *not* be combined with it. There are also recent reports that while Eskimos, whose diet is rich in EPA, have a very low rate of heart disease, they do have a somewhat high rate of strokes. We are not yet sure if there is any connection. If you think EPA pills might be for you, take them under the supervision of your own doctor. Fish oil, even in capsule form, is high in calories. So if you use it as a supplement you may have to cut other calories out of your diet to maintain an ideal rejuvenation weight.

There are other, somewhat miscellaneous supplements that might interest you. *Activated charcoal* has recently been found to lower cholesterol and is now available in tablet form. A newly discovered enzyme called *co-enzyme-Q*, an enzyme our body needs in order to control the flow of oxygen within individual cells, has shown striking results in use with heart disease patients, strengthening the heart muscle (as well as other muscles in the body). *Wheat grass* and *barley grass,* while not yet proven, are believed to have an anti-cancer effect, much the same as cruciferous vegetables, and are available now as a supplement. There are no official dosages yet on any of these new items, so I can only recommend that you use them with caution and under the supervision of your physician. One dosage I can strongly recommend, however, is two tablespoons of an acidophilus liquid or powder per day. This mixture, much the same as yogurt, fills our intestines with friendly bacteria, aiding in digestion.

GUIDELINES FOR BUYING AND USING YOUR SUPPLEMENTS

Supplements may cost anywhere from thirty to sixty dollars per month, depending primarily on how many of the amino acids and/or EPA capsules you choose to try. This may, at first, seem like a great investment, but in fact it is probably the least expensive form of health insurance available. I am always quick to remind my patients that any expense incurred for the cause of preventive medicine, if weighed against any kind of medical therapy or treatment, is a bargain second to none. This does not mean that the best supplements are the most expensive, or that you shouldn't try to get the most supplement for your money, or should avoid getting more supplement than you need. But I do suggest that you stick with name brands, preferably those that have been approved by consumer groups. There are a lot of vitamin companies out there, and not a lot of regulation. We want to be sure we are getting what we think we're getting, and paying a little more for that assurance is well worth it.

In seeking out the best vitamin supplement, do not be impressed with "time released." This is pretty meaningless. Do, however, look for those labeled "hypoallergenic" or those stating that they contain no artificial colors, flavors, fillers, cements, salt, wax, or other potential allergy-producing substances such as milk, rye, wheat, corn, starch, or preservatives. The word "natural" is far less important. In fact, there is no evidence that natural vitamins are any more effective than synthetic ones. When buying mineral supplements, most of the same guidelines apply. *Read the labels.* Don't let health store or vitamin store clerks sell you things you don't need. They are salespersons first, health advisors last. Bring this book or a list of what you need with you so that you will not need to ask their unprofessional advice.

Buying the right calcium and EPA capsules requires special advice:

When buying calcium, do not get the *bone meal* or *dolomite* type or any other containing other minerals. At the very least these other minerals are unnecessary, since you will be getting them from your multimineral and other supplements (and sometimes they contain toxins, like lead); and at worst, some of these minerals may block the absorption of the calcium. For my own patients, I usually recommend calcium carbonate, which usually works out to be the most economical and seems to be equally as effective as the more expensive types.

When buying EPA capsules make sure it is a 300 milligram capsule in a 1000 milligram base and that the base does not contain vitamin A or vitamin D, which may become toxic if taken this way (which is why I do not recommend cod liver oil). Since EPA is relatively new on the market, proper controls are not yet established, and some EPA capsules may contain other undesirable substances, including—believe it or not—cholesterol. Reading labels and asking questions of doctor and salesman are, in this case, essential.

Equally as important as informed buying is informed usage of supplements. Do not refrigerate! Refrigeration destroys vitamins and minerals. As a general rule make sure to take all supplements with food as they are best absorbed along with regular digestion and can irritate an empty stomach. Also, since some supplements help others, while some block the absorption of others, we need to chart a simple schedule to make sure we are getting maximum benefit.

The table below lists some important dynamics of mineral absorption. If we take iron, we need to take it separately from the three minerals which obstruct it, while boosting it with vitamins C and E and copper. Since vitamin C also aids calcium, but calcium blocks iron, we want to divide our vitamin C between these two minerals. Zinc helps copper, and copper helps iron, but zinc blocks iron. This creates a conflict. In cases such as these, the first priority is to avoid allowing any nutrient to get in the way of another. If in the process we are unable to boost a certain nutrient, that is less serious.

MINERAL ABSORPTION INFORMATION

Mineral	**Aided by**
Calcium	vitamin C, EPA fish oil, magnesium, vitamin D, acids
Copper	zinc
Iron	vitamin C, vitamin E, copper
Magnesium	vitamin C, calcium, protein
Zinc	B vitamins, vitamin E

Mineral	**Blocked by**
Iron	calcium, magnesium, zinc
Copper	excess zinc

There are many things I have advised or suggested throughout this chapter which the medical establishment has not yet embraced. If I had written this book ten years ago I would be pointing to things like the importance of zinc, calcium, and magnesium that were, at that time, not popular issues but which are now a part of the status quo. With this in mind I predict that much of what I'm saying now will one day be regarded as good sound medicine. My advice to you is not to wait for that time. When it comes to your vital nutrients, don't wait for the symptoms of a deficiency; make sure, as a preventive measure, that you are getting enough. Throughout this chapter I have mentioned specific vitamins and minerals that can be depleted due to illness or stress; but, in fact, every single nutrient we consume, whether in food or supplement form, can be depleted to a greater or lesser degree by several factors we want to avoid as much as possible: excess saturated fat, excess refined sugars and refined carbohydrates, excess alcohol, unclean water, stress, and excessive use of medication.

I have already dealt with the issues of saturated fat, white paste, and water; stress will be explored in Chapter 6; and in the next chapter, you will discover some startling information on the issue of drugs and their effect on nutrition.

4 The Nutrition-Drug Connection

As time passes, no matter how well we take care of ourselves, nutritionally or otherwise, we may still need for various reasons to employ the benefits of certain medications. While I am never overly anxious to prescribe any drug, I have always recognized that there are many drugs and medications that are invaluable to the cause of preserving, increasing, and enhancing human life. But regardless of their value in fighting illness and suffering, they all have side effects. These side effects are vast and vary in degree. Some are minor in comparison to the importance of the drug; other side effects do us far more harm than the drug does us good. I cannot, in these few pages, possibly discuss all the known side effects of all common medications, but there is one particular kind of side effect that is of particular interest to us if, through following the Rejuvenation Diet, we hope to reverse illness and grow younger. All medications we take interact with the nutrients in our bodies, sometimes to our detriment.

There are two very general ways of looking at nutrient-drug interactions. Once inside the body, nutrients and drugs all break down into their chemical components. The molecules that comprise nutrients can enhance or obstruct the molecules of the medication. This kind of interaction is almost always considered by your physician, who will usually tell you what not to eat with your drugs, so you don't need me to tell you. My job is to make you aware of the effects of drugs on the nutrients we consume. After all, there is not much use in following the Rejuvenation Diet if all our anti-cancer, anti-heart disease, immunity-strengthening nutrients are being strangled and depleted by the medications we are being prescribed. If we are serious about growing and staying younger, we must take measures to make sure we are always getting adequate nutrition.

One universal rule regarding all drug-nutrient interactions is this: never take supplements at the same time as medications. If both must be taken with food, take them at different meals.

The goal of our plan, of course, is to eliminate the need for any and all drugs wherever reasonable and possible. Twenty-three years of practicing medicine tells me that for most people who follow the Rejuvenation Diet along with exercise, an active lifestyle, and the proper frame of mind, those common ailments that are "supposed" to increase with age—chronic headaches, constipation, chest pains, heartburn, backache, depression, insomnia, anxiety attacks, memory loss, immune deficiency illnesses such as infections and arthritis, and any number of other typical symptoms which send people to the medicine chest—will likely start to decrease as you grow younger. There will, however, still be times when certain medications are needed, and a little knowledge can make for safe, if drastically reduced, drug use.

There are three basic ways in which drugs interfere with good nutrition. Some drugs suppress or stimulate the appetite;

others hinder our ability to digest, absorb, and/or metabolize nutrients; still other drugs have a chemical structure so similar to certain nutrients that they travel through the blood stream as partners, and the particular vitamin or mineral is unable to work chemically as it was intended. Multiple drug use, especially if it is chronic or long term, can further complicate nutrition-drug interaction, as can natural changes in the body over time, which affect our ability to metabolize certain medications.

A few years ago a sixty-nine-year-old man was sent to me by his family, who had noticed signs of senility and feared he had Alzheimer's Disease. Upon examining him I discovered he was taking diuretics for high blood pressure, beta-blockers to control an irregular heart rhythm, tranquilizers for anxiety, and a daily dose of an over-the-counter antihistamine for a chronic stuffy nose. All of these drugs, not surprisingly, were making him disoriented, confused, and depressed. Upon examining him, I also discovered that he was very low in magnesium, zinc, and potassium, which is depleted by diuretics. I immediately took him off the tranquilizers, the beta-blockers, and the antihistamine, reduced his dosage of the diuretics, and prescribed the Rejuvenation Diet with vitamin and mineral insurance, a good daily dose of exercise, and a course in biofeedback. Within *three weeks* the man was as sharp as ever.

I do not mean to imply that everyone, or even a majority of people, on drug therapy have been misdiagnosed or are being given drugs that are doing more harm than good; but I do mean to highlight the potential hazards. If you are already on necessary medication for such conditions as diabetes, ulcers, arthritis, high blood pressure, or heart disease, in this chapter I will briefly describe the possible effect of what you are probably taking and tell you what I tell my patients who require such medication, beginning with this advice: have your physician reevaluate your medication needs every three to six months. I have a sign in my waiting room reminding patients to "Bring all medications to your next check up." I do this for a number of reasons, most importantly to reconsider the need for the medication, but also to make sure that the patient is not by accident taking his or her Aunt Sylvia's medicine, or that the pharmacist (they are not perfect) did not make a mistake in prescription or dosage, and to be certain that the patient is complying. Drugs are a double-edged sword. For most every drug benefit there is a potential side effect, and so drugs can make us ill almost as often as they improve us. But we can shift that ratio and make sure that when medications are called for, the drug serves us *without* harming us.

Ask your doctor exactly what the drug he is prescribing is supposed to do, what might be the side effects, and what, if anything, you can do to defend against those side effects. Find out also how long you might have to take this drug, and if there are any alternatives to taking it. The same goes for over-the-counter (OTC) medicines, which account for about half the drugs sold in this country. These drugs are potentially more harmful than prescribed medications since they are mostly used without the supervision of a doctor. Most OTCs, for legal reasons, advise you to consult your physician before taking more than the maximum dosage. But I say consult your physician before taking the *minimum* dosage of *anything* more than a few times. Ask your doctor what impact the drug will have on you nutritionally, and find out if the drugs you purchase contain any potentially harmful additives. Some common drugs contain caffeine, others contain alcohol. Neither substance is beneficial to our health. Other drugs contain "questionable" ingredients. Many physicians would be shocked to learn that a very well-known female hormone medication, for example, used to (and may still) be coated with carnuba wax—the same wax we spread on our automobiles—with the name of the drug written on the tablet in black India ink.

It is, of course, not possible in these pages to advise anyone whether or not to take any medication, nor is it possible to brief you on every single drug on the market. But I can make you aware of the most common nutrient-drug interactions, with some general guidelines regarding what to do about them.

STAY HUNGRY . . . BUT NOT TOO HUNGRY: DRUGS AND APPETITE

A great percentage of medications, prescription or OTC, can cause stomach disturbances, dry and sore mouths, and decreased taste, all of which can, for some people, suppress the appetite or instigate cravings for high-flavor, low-nutrient foods and overeating. Other medications are now known to act directly on the nervous system, increasing or decreasing the desire to eat. All of this can result in nutritional deficiencies as well as obesity and other illnesses.

Over the counter, beware of frequent use of *analgesics* such as *aspirin.* They can upset the stomach, which causes many people to increase food intake (and calories) in an attempt to soothe the discomfort. *Antihistamines* and *antacids* have been found to decrease appetite, which can decrease nutrition. If you use these medications only occasionally, however, there is little to worry about. If you use them habitually, then (as I will later discuss) we need to take a good hard look at why. Diet pills, which are, of course, supposed to depress appetite, do many other things as well: they can cause strokes, heart irregularities, and high blood pressure. They sometimes do depress the appetite but are never a long-term solution to obesity—or vanity. The scientific name for them is phenylpropanolamine; they are known as PPA for short, and I have told more than a few patients to please let PPA stand for "Please Put them Away."

As for prescription drugs, those I call "appetite-altering" drugs fall into five categories. *Antidepressants,* such as tricyclics and lithium, can sometimes cause bloating and bring on cravings for refined sugars, which we now know to deplete important nutrients. *Antianxiety agents,* such as Librium and Valium, will, in low doses, often increase appetite, while higher doses can suppress appetite to dangerous levels. *Antipsychotic agents,* such as lithium carbonate and those of the phenothiazine group, such as chlorpromazine, have been known to stimulate the appetite so much that sudden obesity often results. Many patients trying to recover from cancer have discovered that their appetite loss from the cancer is exacerbated by the *cancer drug therapy* they are on; and certain digitalis preparation *heart medicines,* such as Digoxin (commonly prescribed to increase heart efficiency) can, in high doses, cause nausea, loss of appetite, decreased food intake, and often a protein deficiency (just what a person with heart disease does not need).

In the case of digitalis heart medicines, if loss of appetite occurs while blood levels of digitalis are at normal levels, an extra 10 to 30 milligrams of the B vitamins may help normalize the appetite. Make sure as well to get frequent blood tests to determine whether the medication is still called for or whether the dosage cannot be reduced.

But beyond that, for these and other medications which decrease or increase your appetite, check into any alternatives with your physician. If there is no avoiding the medication and its accompanying side effects for any period of time, make sure you are adequately nourished without overfeeding yourself. For some people this involves writing out a prescriptive diet of nutrient-dense foods and making sure not to fall below or above it, eating temporarily as though food were a prescriptive medicine. The annoyance of such a regimen may help remind us of the need to reevaluate the necessity for the drug. In some cases this can lead, if nothing else, to a changing of the medication until one is found that does not affect appetite as adversely. Medications cannot make us healthy if we allow our eating habits to compromise our health.

A METABOLIC MYSTERY: DRUGS AND MALABSORPTION

Food, in order to fuel us, needs to be absorbed properly; it must be carried through our blood vessels to the liver for processing into energy. If it does not enter the blood vessels, the fuel is useless.

It is not possible for us to detect how much of every food

we eat is properly absorbed and metabolized in our bodies, and there are many potential causes for malabsorption—stress, for example, or even heredity—but we can certainly be aware of the potential hazards of drugs as they relate to this problem. Once they are in our bodies, drugs and foods are broken down into chemicals, many of them very similar. These chemicals must share the same stomach, and thus there is no avoiding their ultimate contact. The chemicals from a drug can change the character of the chemicals in the foods we eat, rendering them unabsorbable, in which case they may be excreted in the form of newly formed, unusable chemicals; or drugs can impair the intestinal tract so that it cannot properly absorb certain nutrients. There are a number of drugs, over-the-counter as well as prescription medications (not to mention alcohol), that are likely to cause malabsorption.

There are three types of OTCs to beware of in this context. *Antacids,* especially when taken at mealtime, can neutralize the stomach to the point where there is not enough left for normal absorption of folacin. This can trigger a deficiency of the folic acid needed to manufacture blood cells, resulting in an anemia. Antacids containing aluminum, such as Rolaids, Mylanta, Gelusil, Digel, Maalox, Wingel, Aludrox, and Kolantyl, can potentially severely compromise our ability to absorb calcium, increasing the risk of osteoporosis and other bone diseases. Antacids can also decrease the body's ability to absorb vitamin B-12. If you use antacids occasionally, don't worry. The effect will be minute. If you use them every day, this need should probably cease once the Rejuvenation Diet is a part of your life. If you still insist on habitual use of this drug, then have your physician check you for a deficiency of calcium and B-12.

Another group of OTC drugs to watch out for are the common phenolphthalein *laxatives,* such as Ex-lax, Alophen, and Feen-a-mint, as well as the laxatives made from senna, such as Senokot or Dulcolax. All of these can compromise our calcium metabolism, as well as our ability to absorb all the B vitamins. A recent study conducted in England found that the stimulator chemical panthron—contained in most laxatives (Modane, Doxidan, and Dorbantyl to name a few) can cause liver and colon cancer. Another popular laxative which must be used with caution is mineral oil, which may stop the absorption of fat-soluble vitamins A (and beta carotene), D, E, and K. The mineral oil washes these important nutrients right out of the body before they can be absorbed in the blood stream. Once you begin your rejuvenation program of healthy eating and living habits, which includes high fiber, lots of fluids, exercise, and decreased stress, you will never need another laxative again; but if for some reason you do need a laxative on an ongoing basis, make sure your doctor checks you for the potential deficiencies.

Painkillers may also block nutrient absorption. Aspirin and any of the acetaminophen or anti-inflammatory medications like Azulfidine or Indomethacin and Ibuprofen, commonly taken by people suffering from arthritis, cramps, muscle aches and pains, and colitis and headaches, can cause deficiencies in vitamin C, folic acid, and iron. So if it takes a while for good eating, exercise, and a healthy outlook on life to eliminate such chronic (or at least recurring) pain, and if the pain gets so excruciating that you need the temporary relief of a drug, make sure your daily supplement program includes at least my recommended dosage of vitamin C and folic acid to insure against a deficiency. Also have your doctor keep an eye on your iron level to determine if it is necessary for you to take an extra iron supplement; and if so, take it two to three hours before or after any painkiller, other drug, or other supplement.

Prescription drugs that may block the absorption of nutrients are numerous. *Antibiotics,* such as tetracyclines, can cause a number of nutritionally adverse reactions in the body. As they kill invading bacteria in our bodies, they can also kill our important intestinal bacteria. This can severely decrease the amount of folacin, potentially resulting in anemia. Whenever a patient of mine has to be on one of these medications for an extended period of time I always prescribe an acidophilus preparation. This is a liquid solution of lactobacillus acidophilus full of friendly bacteria needed in our intestines. Lowfat yogurt, also containing these friendly bacteria, should also work. I also make sure to monitor iron levels in case I might have to prescribe additional iron-rich foods and an iron supplement. If your doctor discovers that you need to pay closer attention to your iron intake while on these antibiotics, take your iron, be it from food or supplement sources, at least *three hours before* or *three hours after* taking the drug.

Other antibiotics, such as Gentamicin, can cause a deficiency of magnesium, while other antibiotics, taken over long periods of time can interfere with the absorption of calcium. Another class of drugs known as *steroids,* such as estrogens and progesterones often taken by postmenopausal women, can bring on the same problem if taken over long periods of time. Other drugs that interfere with calcium absorption are *cortisones,* such as prednisone, used for a variety of arthritic diseases, skin diseases, blood and lung diseases, allergies, tumors, and neurological disorders, and the *anticonvulsants* phenobarbital and Dilantin. Drugs that might get in the way of magnesium metabolism include colchicine, an *antigout medicine* and *anti-inflammatory chemical,* and a number of *diuretics,* which are prescribed to cause the removal of body water. If it is necessary for you to take any drug that might hinder your ability to absorb calcium or magnesium, make sure to protect your bones by eating the nutrient-dense Rejuvenation Diet, along with vitamin and mineral supplement insurance. If you are already doing that, you need not worry, though you should probably have your magnesium level checked by your doctor to determine whether extra magnesium is called for.

Another serious side effect of some diuretics, such as thiazides, is their interference with fat and glucose metabolism. Over time, these drugs can actually raise LDL—"bad guy" cholesterol—as well as raising blood triglyceride levels, so that in some cases this drug, which is prescribed to decrease the risk of heart disease, can actually *increase* that very risk. If you have to take these diuretics, you may have to significantly decrease your cholesterol intake, perhaps to less than 300 milligrams per day (which is below normal rejuvenation levels) and, under a doctor's supervision, take some extra niacin.

The *anti-cholesterol drugs* Questran and Colestid, quickly becoming popular prescribed treatments for high cholesterol, can hinder our ability to absorb vitamins A, D, E, K, and folic acid. With patients of mine whose LDL cholesterol is at such a dangerously high level that we cannot safely wait for the effects of proper eating, exercise, and a new frame of mind to lower it, I feel that I must prescribe one of these medications, but I always make sure that they increase their supplemental dosages to 10,000 IUs of beta carotene, 400 IUs of D, 1 milligram of folic acid per day, and *under the observation of a doctor,* 2 to 25 milligrams of K. (Never take vitamin K unless monitored by your physician; it can imbalance clotting mechanisms if taken in excess).

THE GREAT PRETENDER: WHEN DRUGS MIMIC NUTRIENTS

Some drugs have a chemical structure so similar to certain nutrients that they travel through the blood stream hooked to one another, and the particular vitamin or mineral, even though it has been successfully absorbed into the blood stream, is still unable to do its job for us.

There are a great many prescription medicines that can mimic, and therefore obstruct our body's use of, several of the B-vitamins. *Tranquilizers,* such as Mellaril, Stelazine, and Thorazine, can cheat us out of our B-2, so if it is imperative that we take these tranquilizers we should also take a minimum of 5 extra milligrams of vitamin B-2 per day.

Many other medicines can get in the way of our B-6. These include *antihypertensive medicines,* such as Apresoline; *cortisone* drugs, such as Medrol and Deltasone; *estrogen* drugs such as Premarin; *anti-Parkinson disease drugs,* such as L-Dopa; and birth control pills. If you absolutely need an antihypertension drug, you'll likely need 25 extra milligrams of B-6 per day. If you're on birth control pills for any reason, 5 to 10 extra milligrams of B-6 per day should cover your needs; and add to that 0.4 to 1 microgram of folic acid. Some drugs that antagonize our potential supply of vitamin B-12 and folic acid are the *antibiotics* Achromycin, Macrodantin, Septra, Sumycin, and Bactrim (commonly prescribed to treat bladder and urinary infections); the *antihypertensive medication* Aldoril; the *diuretic* Dyazide; *cortisone drugs,* such as Deltasone and Medrol; the *pain reliever,* Percodan; the *tranquilizer,* Stelazine; Tagamet, an *anti-ulcer medication;* Premarin, an *estrogen preparation;* and the *stomach medicine* Donnatal. To counteract these counter-nutritional side effects I suggest an extra 100 to 500 milligrams of B-12 and 1 microgram extra of folic acid.

THERE MUST BE A BETTER WAY

There are probably more aspirin junkies in America today than there are alcoholics. The reason that laxatives, antacids, sleeping pills, tranquilizers, and diet pills can all be addictive is that they treat symptoms and not the physical or psychological root cause of the problem. These symptoms are often a sign to us that we must alter our way of living, not an indication that we need to open the medicine cabinet.

The next time you get a tension headache (commonly known as a muscle contraction headache)—and most headaches are from tension—rather than reaching for the aspirin try a little ice on the forehead, or try loosely and slowly rotating your head around in both directions, as taught in hatha yoga. If that doesn't relieve the tension that's causing the headache, try a back and neck massage. With the thumb and forefinger of one hand find the two prominences or knobs at the back of the head—right where the neck connects to the scalp—drop the fingers right below the knobs to the muscle and compress very tightly with both fingers; then with the thumb of the other hand press the point where your nose meets the forehead; and see if this often successful form of accupressure doesn't get rid of your headache in a matter of minutes.

The next time constipation strikes, try three extra glasses

of water and a thirty-minute walk. Drink more water and you will probably find you have less nasal congestion and don't need that antihistamine. If you still have chronic sinus problems, consider the possibility that it might be an allergy or too much steam heat, and bear in mind that it is normal for a human being to produce about two cups of mucus per day—which should not call for a constant drying blast of antihistamine. And the next time you get indigestion from overeating or eating too fast, instead of reaching for relief, start considering a change in the ferocity of your food intake.

Read on, and you will discover how regular exercise, without any negative side effects, can eliminate many of these seemingly chronic conditions, removing the need for those "crutch-type" drugs; and how vigorous daily activity ensures optimum health so that the prescriptive medications we do need to take can give us the greatest benefit.

5 Use It or Lose It: Keeping the Body and Mind Active

There are many good reasons to exercise, and lots of enjoyable and safe ways to go about it. Exercising does not mean breaking your back or twisting your ankle. In fact, for the vast majority of active people, it means the complete opposite. Those who use their muscles and joints are going to be more limber and thus far less likely to suffer such injuries than those people who avoid the slightest strain. This is so for anyone at any age. Even modified exercise in the elderly and the very ill delivers immediate and major results.

The same is true of the mind. The more the brain is challenged, the more it can grow. Exercise of body and mind is part of the prevention and cure for many things: insomnia, depression, constipation, gastrointestinal illness, obesity, high blood pressure, high cholesterol, and heart disease. It can help control diabetes and is a major part of the prevention of senility and many forms of cancer. Exercise is vital to a strong immune system, and ultimately—and most important to everyone who passes through my office through these pages—what all of these benefits add up to is that daily activity of body and mind can help us grow younger, enjoy life more fully, and live much longer. There are many books and doctors recommending exercising less than every day, claiming the body needs repair. I do not buy this argument. Life is motion; life does not take a holiday, and nothing in nature functions while standing still; why should we be any different?

Until only a few decades ago, many physicians believed that exercise delivered no health benefits. (There are still some physicians today who dispute the benefits of exercise, but fortunately they are in the minority.) There was much doubt over whether activity had any relation to obesity, and many in the medical profession even believed that vigorous exercise did permanent damage to the body. Today most of us know better.

We know that exercise increases serotonin, a neurotransmitter (message carrier) in the brain without which we are likely to be depressed and unlikely to get a good night's sleep. Daily exercise can combat depression and insomnia in other ways. It can help us look better, raising self-esteem and making us feel more alive. And the more active we are the more deeply we will sleep, not only because of the increased serotonin in the brain but simply because the human body needs to expend a day's worth of energy in order to feel the need for truly deep and restful sleep.

We also know that lack of body movement, particularly movement of the abdominal muscles, causes constipation in many people. I have seen literally hundreds of patients cure constipation and other irritable bowel syndromes with just a forty-minute daily walk. Continuous movement, it seems, is needed for the abdominal muscles to massage the intestines, causing normal rapid emptying. But a trip to the toilet is not all you will get from a good walk, run, or bike ride.

Exercise dilates the blood vessels, increasing circulation and thus reducing blood pressure. It also lowers blood pressure by reducing body weight, relieving emotional stress, and burning "pressure-producing" chemicals in the body. As we exercise we make the heart a more efficient and stronger muscle. We increase the amount of energy burned, metabolizing more fat, lowering harmful LDL cholesterol, and increasing protective HDL cholesterol. All of this prevents heart disease. In fact, recent studies comparing exercisers to nonexercisers and persons with active jobs (postal delivery workers, longshoremen) to those with sedentary jobs (desk workers and bus drivers) found that people who live life on their feet, using their muscles, are less than *half* as likely to get a heart attack or to die from heart disease—or cancer, for that matter. This comes as no surprise to me, and probably not to you, as it is certainly no secret that a healthy exercise program is necessary to combat obesity, a primary culprit in heart disease. Active people burn far more calories than people who lead sedentary lives.

Lying down or sleeping, for example, uses about 80 calories per hour. Sitting at a desk or in front of a television burns only 100 calories per hour. Clean the house and you're up to about 180 calories per hour; walk two and a half miles and you can burn more than 200 calories; or bike five and a half miles with similar results. Swimming burns 300-plus calories per hour, as does vigorous dancing, tennis, even table tennis. Start running ten miles per hour and you're burning 900 calories per hour. Increase the intensity of any of these or other activities and you increase the body's fuel consumption and improve the body's cardiovascular system. But that's not all. The active person burns calories two to three times more quickly than the nonactive person, even at times during the day when he or she is not doing the exercise. The body, it seems, responds to a good workout by preparing for the next big expenditure of energy, and it does so by burning fuel at a more rapid rate. If you have ever tried to lose weight without exercising, you've probably experienced the opposite effect. The sedentary body, receiving fewer calories, goes into a storage phase and becomes more efficient with its use of calories; it continually stores fat, and you don't lose much weight. Ultimately, all the nutritional knowledge in the world and the best intentions aren't going to make you much healthier without exercise.

By now I hope I have partially convinced the armchair

lovers among you to give this life-sustaining act a try, so let's look at exercise from a positive point of view. Exercise not only burns up calories but can also help us eat less. Many studies have found that a robust workout decreases appetite. This may not seem apparent in many people, myself and some of my patients included, because we almost always exercise before a meal and therefore are naturally hungry. There may also be psychological factors, leading us to believe that we *should* be hungry after working up a sweat. But even so, many of my patients tell me that even when they are very hungry before exercising, their appetite may be diminished so that they will eat less. Other patients who are underweight and have lack-of-appetite problems often find exercise makes them hungry, leading me to believe that for many people vigorous activity seems to regulate the appetite to its ideal state. But perhaps most important of all, I find that my active patients tend not to crave so much junk food. Put this all together and it becomes clear that the number one cause of obesity (which may be the number one cause of heart disease and many types of cancer) is the sedentary life that so many people find themselves unnecessarily leading.

Probably the main cause of cancer, which is cigarette smoking, can also be reversed through exercise. In a random study done a short time ago, researchers found that less than 5 percent of all serious exercisers smoked cigarettes, and that of those who had previously been addicted to tobacco, 81 percent of the men and 76 percent of the women had quit since they started to exercise regularly. Another recent study linking exercise to cancer prevention found that men who worked in jobs requiring no physical activity, who did not have a regular exercise program to compensate, had a *30 percent greater* chance of contracting colon cancer than their more active counterparts. Recent studies show a firm connection between a strong immune system and regular exercise. It has been established that exercise enhances our lymphocytes and our granulocytes, body cells in the blood which strengthen our ability to fight off viruses and bacteria, as well as many forms of cancer.

Other studies, looking in general at longevity without

considering cause of death, found that a lifestyle of eight hours of sitting at a desk followed by six hours on a sofa followed by eight hours in a bed does not enhance longevity. Life insurance companies now try to encourage their policyholders to exercise because they know that active people overwhelmingly tend to live longer and better than inactive people. This doesn't mean we have to change our careers in order to increase our life expectancy; it simply means that we have to make exercise a part of our leisure time (though, in fact, as I will later explain, you can even do aerobic exercise sitting at your desk). A recent study found that regular exercise expends about 3500 calories per week, resulting in half the risk of death as those who do not exercise; further research suggests that a lifetime of exercise may even reduce the negative effects of years of cigarette smoking, high blood pressure, and offset any inherited tendency toward early death.

The benefits of exercise are wide-ranging, and many of them are no longer secret to most people. Yet it is doubtful that science and medicine know *all* the benefits of a life that includes vigorous and intelligent exercise. I, for example, who keep up on every study citing every benefit, only recently discovered a study of several years ago demonstrating that physical training increased tissue sensitivity to insulin in proportion to the degree of improved physical fitness. This indicates that *exercise alone* may play a major role in managing adult-onset diabetes mellitus. Of course, I was already convinced that exercise is a vital and basic human need. I hope that now you are, too.

EXERCISE DOESN'T HAVE TO BE A PAIN IN THE NECK

Many of us were brought up to hate exercise. Bad early experiences with gym class can explain much of this: embarrassment and humiliation on the playing field, then being punished for misbehaving by running laps around the field or gym. Now some doctor is also telling you to take laps. Only this time it's to improve and prolong your life, and you don't have to run; I am a great proponent of walking.

There are many ways to exercise, none of which has to include the thrill of victory, the agony of defeat, or the agony of a wrenched back; and there are many good books (some of which are recommended in the back of this book) suggesting fun and adventurous ways to go about it—if you're into fun and adventure. But you don't have to be. Regular physical activity should not be confused with vigorous athletic training, which in recent studies was found to be less positive for longevity than a lifetime commitment to moderate exercise. All you need to know is how to be sure it is aerobic.

Aerobic exercise must use large muscle groups, it must be rhythmical, and it must be done continuously. Here are a few examples of aerobic exercise, including my favorites, which I will elaborate on in the following sections: swimming, biking (moving or stationary), brisk walking, aerobic dancing, rowing, cross-country skiing (outdoors or on cross-country skiing machines), and jogging.

The effectiveness of any aerobic exercise is determined by three factors: frequency, duration, and intensity.

Frequency for me means five to seven times a week. While some experts contend that more than five times a week offers no additional cardiovascular benefits, the other exercise benefits have not been found to reach any kind of plateau. Besides, I find the mental and emotional benefits of exercise so valuable I cannot imagine intentionally letting a day go by without breaking some kind of a sweat. Some of you may prefer to mix aerobic exercise with flexibility-type exercise, such as hatha yoga, which also raises the heart rate considerably and which I will elaborate on later in this chapter. When exercise is a daily habit, it vastly decreases the possibility that we might think up an excuse not to exercise; and when unforeseen circumstances prevent us on a given day from exercising, we'll probably be eager to pick up where we left off. Exercising less than five times a week produces minimal benefits; however, we must be careful not to allow exercise to become a destructive addiction, increasing it beyond what is healthy, or putting it between us and our personal relationships.

Duration means how long we exercise each time. For me,

twenty minutes is the absolute minimum, and a good place to start for those of you for whom it has been a while. With time, you'll find yourself up to thirty minutes. Our ideal goal is an hour a day.

Intensity refers to the increase in our heart rate during exercise. The simplest way to monitor your active heart rate is to take your wrist pulse for six seconds, while exercising, and multiply it by ten. An advisable intensity is from 60 to 80 percent of your heart's maximum capacity. (Some still recommend up to 90 percent, which I consider a bit much and potentially dangerous unless you are in peak physical condition.) The easiest way to compute your maximum heart rate is to subtract your age from 220 as shown below:

BEATS PER MINUTE

Age	Maximum rate	60% rate	80% rate
35	185	111	148
40	180	108	144
45	174	105	140
50	170	102	136
55	165	99	132
60	160	96	128
65	155	93	124
70	150	90	120
75	145	87	116
80	140	84	112
85	135	81	108
90	130	78	104
95	125	75	100
100	120	72	96
105	115	69	92
110	110	66	89

No matter how healthy you think you are right now, it is wise for anyone beginning an exercise program to get a medical examination. In trying to improve the heart muscle there is always the possibility, if we are not under some kind of medical supervision, that we could overdo it. We've all heard stories about fifty or forty or even thirty-year-olds who decide to correct all the years of inactivity in one afternoon, with dire consequences. Even athletes, and their coaches, have been known to push themselves into coronaries. One visit to a responsible physician can usually remove most danger from your new commitment to an active life.

If you feel you are at something less than peak physical condition, go easy on yourself, but be demanding; make sure you increase duration and intensity as you get into better shape. If you are already involved with running or swimming, that's great. Or if you have a fondness for any particular aerobic activity (or a combination of a few) that you wouldn't mind engaging in five to seven times a week, that's wonderful. Do it! If exercise is new for you, that is not a disadvantage. In fact, I have found that often the patients who were great athletes in their youth, accustomed to hearing cheers and applause as reward for their efforts, can sometimes lack the self-motivation of those of you who have come to understand the most important reasons to exercise. Many people like to combine exercise with social activity: walking, running, tennis partners. Engaging in competitive sports, however, may produce more stress and anxiety than the workout itself relieves. I personally enjoy an occasional game of tennis with a sportsmanlike opponent, though I do not make it a regular part of my exercise program. Following are my three favorite ways to exercise my body. One of them is aerobic, one of them is the flexibility type, and one of them is purely for enjoyment.

The Best Advice You'll Ever Get: Take a Walk

No one is ever too old to walk, and a brisk forty to sixty-minute walk does as much for our cardiovascular system as the same amount of any other exercise. In fact, recent studies have found that people who walk regularly at a pace of 5.5 miles per hour or more are in the top one percent of cardiovascular fitness. Walking one mile in fifteen minutes burns the same number of calories as jogging an equal distance in 8.5 minutes. Heavier people who walk burn even more calories. By moving the arms vigorously while walking we can increase its aerobic benefits, and, when we feel we are ready, we can challenge ourselves with upgrades, stairs, even hills. Walking can be done alone or with others, and without special equipment, just comfortable shoes or sneakers and comfortable clothes. With very little risk of injury, walking can be done any time, day or night, at sunrise or during your lunch hour. One of my patients is an attorney who works down the street from my office. For years he claimed he was too busy to exercise; now I see him walking away his lunch hour, giving out dictation to his secretary (who may one day be grateful to him for the exercise) as she walks beside him. This man may not receive the relaxation benefits of his activity, but at least he is strengthening his heart and keeping fit. Other patients of mine have tried this excuse: "There's no place in Los Angeles (or New York or Chicago) that's safe to walk in. . . ." Nonsense! I send such complainers to the nearest indoor shopping mall, preferably early in the day, before it gets too crowded. I have recently learned that during the winter in many cities whole groups of people meet in malls to do their daily walking. Just make sure you do not stop to browse. Walking for exercise must be continuous—that means uninterrupted—in order to be aerobic. Walking the dog, therefore, may present a problem (though a well-trained dog, I have discovered, will keep up with your pace for your hour of exercise, then, when you are through, take care of his business). Walking is turning into a major cultural trend, with entire books (some of which I recommend in the back of this book) and magazines devoted to its pursuit, and full of the latest information about stretching before and cooling off after a brisk walk so as to get the maximum benefit without risking injury. If you have any doubt what kind of exercise program to take up, I urge you to do what comes naturally to all of us: Do some relaxing warm-ups, stretching and bending, then hold your head up, back straight, tuck in your abdomen, and take a walk.

Meditation in Motion

All exercise relieves stress to some degree but in my opinion none does so as much as hatha yoga. The stretching and movement involved in yoga are extremely invigorating. Yoga burns calories, improves coordination, and makes us more limber than ever, so that we can avoid pulled muscles and strained tendons in our other exercise. While it may not be classically aerobic, it is in many other ways one of the most complete workouts we can give ourselves, and it also induces a state of relaxation by inducing alpha brain wave relaxation and vastly increasing brain serotonin. Yoga teaches breathing techniques that can enable us to control stress and anxiety and induce calm—without tranquilizers!—at any time. In a world full of countless and unavoidable stresses and anxieties, this means a lot to me. I have often prescribed hatha yoga to my patients and radio listeners, not only as part of an aerobic exercise program but also as part of a stress-management plan. You can find a yoga studio in the Yellow Pages or try the easy-to-follow instructions in Choudhury and Reynold's book, *Bikram's Beginning Yoga.* I recommend yoga three times a week for one to one and a half hours; and if you think it's a breeze, check your heart rate after your first session.

Sexercise

Someone once said: "Sex doesn't make you live longer, it only makes you want to live longer." But active sex does burn large numbers of calories, decreasing the risk of obesity and its related illnesses; and sex certainly increases the heartbeat. I am not suggesting that anyone should set up a rigid schedule of sexual activity, or in any way compromise spontaneity, but I think it is important to point out all of its benefits—which are true for anyone at any age. It is pretty well established now that an active sex life can drastically reduce a man's chances of developing cancer of the prostate; and there is no question that sex can induce relaxation and calm and that it helps to satisfy our crucial need for human touch, caring, and intimacy, all of which are basic needs that are linked directly to the integrity of our immune system—not to mention our psyche and soul. So sex may, after all, prove to be helpful in increasing longevity. Our society no longer disapproves of us enjoying sex after our reproductive years. In fact, more and more studies are finding that for a vast number of people, lovemaking gets better with the passage of time. The Kinsey Report and hundreds of other studies since have established that sexual interest need not decline with age. Furthermore, as we grow our lives change, making acts of love easier to engage in (post menopausal women need not worry about contraceptives; and as our children begin to leave the nest—or at least stay away from it for extended periods of time—privacy is much easier to come by). Finally, according to Dr. Robert Butler of the Mount Sinai School of Medicine in New York City, as we get older we get better at lovemaking (and, of course, we get slower, which in the case of making love is always better).

Admittedly, many people's sex lives have much room for improvement. Over the years I have had many patients confide in me about their sexual dilemmas, their fear of becoming impotent or frigid. The physician-patient relationship is a very personal one, and for people who are somewhat detached from their spouse—or divorced or widowed—and are not seeing a therapist, I am the only person with whom they feel they can share such problems. I, of course, never trained as a sex therapist, but I consider it my duty as a doctor to help whenever possible; and experience in this role has taught me a lot of what needs to be said.

Most people simply have to learn to defy the myth that sex after a certain age is impossible, silly, a waste of time, or something that "older people" (whatever that means) don't do. Ironically, for some people this mythical age of mandatory celibacy is fifty; for others it is as much as eighty or ninety—

though not a bit more valid. In fact, the main reason a person can lose his or her sex drive at a certain age is that he or she decides, for whatever reason, to stop having sex. As with every other part of the human body, if you don't use it you are likely to lose it. This goes for the genitals and every other erogenous zone, especially those in the brain.

There are other reasons for sexual dormancy. Hostility, fear of intimacy, frigidity, and impotence (which, although often psychological, can also be caused by excessive alcohol, tobacco, and many over-the-counter medicines, especially antihistamines). And for many people, finding a sexual partner is no simple matter.

Since I am not a sex therapist, a marriage counselor, or a dating coach, the only advice I can really offer is this: don't give up. By growing younger and adding a few decades to your life, you'll have more time to pursue an active sex life. You'll also have more energy; energy encourages our sex drive and makes us more attractive; and an active sex life in turn increases the energy we have for other aspects of our lives. And finally, what rejuvenation gives us toward satisfying all of our physical and emotional needs is that most precious commodity: self-worth.

Chairbound Aerobics

I once had a patient who, after taking a sixty-mile-an-hour spill on a motorcycle, found himself paralyzed from the waist down. He told me he had decided very early on in his recuperation not to feel sorry for himself and not to let his life be any less enjoyable because of his handicap. He remained careful about his diet and maintained a positive attitude toward his future, but he worried that his confinement and lack of exercise might diminish his muscle tone and might in the long run shorten his life. Having never been posed this dilemma before, I was at a loss, but the man's courage and optimism inspired me to find him an answer. There is, it turns out, no reason a person cannot get a full aerobic workout without relying on any part of the lower body. There are a number of exercises done with the upper body that can easily increase the heartbeat to 80 percent and increase our metabolic rate as well as tone up the upper portion of the body.

Here are just a few examples, all of them to be done for as long as possible, using the same heart rate schedule as for any other exercise:

> Extend the arms all the way out and twirl them in tight six-inch circles, forward and backward, up to and maintaining maximum speed.
>
> Swing the arms up and down, as in jumping jacks.
>
> Swing the arms in front and behind, as fast as you can, for a sustained period of time.
>
> Lift shoulders up, around, and down with rapidly increasing intensity.

After a while, my paraplegic friend started adding two and then five-pound weights to increase the intensity of his workout. You may want to try this with the supervision of your doctor.

Since prescribing these exercises for my paraplegic friend, I have discovered that they are also ideal for people who break a leg or sprain an ankle, or for people who are at times confined to a desk for ten hours a day. Though I do not recommend these as a permanent exercise program for anyone with leg mobility, they can be a wonderful addition when done during a daily walk.

Another wonderful exercise, though not yet proven to be classically aerobic but which can be done sitting or standing, is singing. It has been found to be excellent for developing breath control, reducing asthma, and increasing blood circulation; and best of all it's fun and relieves stress.

"Brainrobics": Exercising the Mind

According to the National Institute on Aging, only a miniscule number of brain cells diminish because of aging. The only proven causes of brain deterioration are chemical abuse of alcohol or other mood-altering drugs, and lack of use.

Patients of mine have complained of losing their memory—especially when they miss an appointment. I remember quite vividly one woman of forty-eight sitting on an examining table and exclaiming with a sense of defeat, "I guess I'm just getting older."

"What is it you can't remember?" I asked.

She shrugged. "I write everything down because I'm sure I'll forget, and then I can't remember where I wrote it. . . ." She had even tried writing down where she had put her list of things to remember; and then, of course, she would forget where that list was, and so on. In her effort to avoid having to rely on her brain to remember anything, she had undermined her ability to remember, not to mention the belief in herself that she could.

I "prescribed" a number of memory exercises, brain teasers, and crossword puzzles—not that she needed to *improve* her memory, just to *use* it—and within a few months she did not feel so old and forgetful anymore.

Other patients think they're losing their mind because they can't add a few simple numbers together (usually they're checking my bill) until I find out why they can't add anymore: they've been using a calculator to add for them for the last twelve years. It is not a terribly profound idea, but if you stop doing something long enough there is a good chance you will forget how to do it. How many of us forgot the foreign language we learned in high school because we never used it again? The cure, of course, is to get back on the metaphorical horse: throw away your calculator, if need be, and require yourself to remember more; you may be surprised how much you are, and have always been, capable of storing in your head. Many of my patients who think they are losing their mind with age, however, are merely noticing more of the shortcomings that were always there. I think the most absent-minded group of humans I have ever encountered are teenagers. Are adolescents senile? Is their grey matter deteriorating? Or are they just preoccupied?

There are illnesses that bring on the appearance of senility: hypothyroidism and other endocrine illnesses, anemia, diabetes, malnutrition, chronic infections, lung disease, tumors, drug reactions, and even severe vitamin deficiencies. But perhaps one of the most common causes of a person's "losing" his or her mind over time is that he or she was not *using* his or her mind. We shouldn't allow ourselves to become bored or depressed to the point of sensory deprivation. Keep reading, keep writing (letters, a diary, stories), balance your checkbook without a machine, do brain teasers if they amuse you, discuss the meaning of life with a six-year-old—whatever. A healthy diet will help. So will daily physical exercise. Just keep the juices flowing and they will never dry up.

Make It Second Nature: An Active Mindset

Once you begin to experience the benefits of exercise—the physical well-being, improved appearance, raised self-worth, increased energy, and relaxation—make it more than just that daily hour commitment. Don't wait for the elevator; choose the stairs. (Do this within reason; consult your doctor before climbing more than one or two flights at a time.) The next time you drive to the movies and the parking lot is full, don't panic. Don't get angry at the guy who stole the last parking space from you. He did you a favor. He gave you a chance to park a few blocks away and get in a brief walk. Next time you go to the movies, don't even try to park in the lot. Take a walk. If you play golf, sell your golf cart. If you have a lawn, mow it yourself with a hand-operated mower (provided your doctor has approved it for you). It all adds up to a longer and healthier life.

6 Completing the Approach: Your Mental/Emotional/Spiritual "Supplement"

At this point in medical history, no rejuvenation plan could possibly be complete without addressing itself to the mind-body connection. The human body and mind are not separate entities. They do not function independently of each other. In fact, they do not function at all without each other. Hippocrates realized this a few thousand years ago, but since then and until very recently medicine and technology have completely ignored these profound ideas. The evidence, however, has been mounting for about six to eight years now, and even the most conservative sectors of the medical establishment have begun to consider that the way we feel emotionally has a major influence, short-term as well as long-term, on our physical state and in many cases on our life expectancy. For more than fifty years we have accepted that ulcers are largely emotional in origin. Now it seems more than likely that a myriad of other illnesses, including heart disease, cancer, and all other immune deficiency syndromes can be exacerbated or intensified by years of stress, anger, anxiety, depression, and hopelessness. Even cholesterol can be greatly influenced by our moods. I have seen patients who followed a low-fat, high-fiber diet along with a rigorous daily exercise program and still had dangerously high cholesterol; it was purely stress-induced.

Looking at these important findings from a positive point of view, what they tell us is that now we may very well have a much firmer grasp on how to prevent, or even reverse, all of these conditions. If we can simply improve our emotional life, we will not only make life more pleasurable but we will make it healthier and probably make it last a lot longer. We must not, of course, rule out emotional syndromes as being possible *symptoms* of illness; severe depression, for example, is the first symptom, usually occurring about eighteen months before the actual onset, of pancreatic cancer. But depression and other emotional problems are most often the cause and not the result of some physical sickness, and so they must be taken seriously as a major health concern.

Psychosomatic illness is no longer an obscure psychiatric disorder. It is very common, and mostly undiagnosed. Perhaps the most common reason is that many people, not surprisingly, connect illness with receiving kindness, attention, love. I was once referred a forty-eight-year-old woman with chronic debilitating headaches. She had been to over a dozen doctors and had neither found the cause nor the cure for her condition. After examining her and finding no physical maladies, I simply asked: "Why do you want this headache?" She glared at me as if I were crazy. She told me I was crazy. Then she turned away, started to cry, and out poured this reminiscence: she was nine years old, her parents were leaving the house, leaving her alone; she was afraid they weren't ever coming back; she got a severe headache and cried and held her head, and her parents took her with them. Ever since then she had used this headache to keep people from leaving her. (At the time of her visit to me, it turned out, her daughter was planning to go 3000 miles away to college.) It seemed so obvious to her as she confronted this reality, yet the headaches had been going on so long they had taken on a life of their own. She was no longer in control of them; they were now in control of her. At the time she was not ready for my help, or for anyone's. It wasn't until several years and one good therapist later that she became willing to give up control over people, and give up her agonizing headaches. I have since read a number of reports in medical and health journals documenting other similar cases where the treatment of a headache was only as successful as the patient allowed it to be. In one case, as reported by neurologist Oliver Sacks, when a man was cured of his migraines through medication he quickly developed asthma.

This is not to imply that all—or even most—headaches or asthma attacks are self-inflicted; but it is a possibility that must always be considered. The same can be true of any number of illnesses we may think we are victims of, including heart attacks. We may not even understand our own motive for subjecting ourselves to such sickness, but if we are to stay healthy and rejuvenated, it is a good idea to begin to respect the incredible power of our own minds.

I am not a psychologist, yet twenty-three years of internal medicine have required me to develop an insight into the human psyche so that I can identify when the root cause of an illness is emotional, and my experience has led me to believe that a major resource for the prevention and treatment of almost all common ailments is within our minds. In this chapter, we'll explore some specific mind-body connections made through studies or witnessed in my medical practice, plus some tips on how to deal with them. Obviously, I cannot address every kind of emotional problem that might become an obstacle to rejuvenation, nor can I offer clinical advice. Many emotional issues are too complex to handle in any kind of book. But awareness in these matters is worth its weight in leather couch. Self-esteem is the first step toward solving any personal dilemma; and if you have made a commitment to yourself to follow a rejuvenating diet with daily exercise, then you already possess a measurable amount of self-esteem.

YOUTH IS NOT A NUMBER

Every day it seems that I see a new patient, usually around the age of forty, who suddenly thinks life is a downhill course from now on. If he has not achieved his lifetime goals he now believes that he never will. If she hasn't yet bicycled through France or seen the Great Wall of China, she is sure that time has run out on her. To those who experience it, these feelings are real, they are painful, and they can be dangerous.

Just last week, I saw a man who complained of feeling tired, weak, and short of breath. He thought he might have asthma. He did not. Nor did he have any illness that could be diagnosed through medical tests. I told him he was in great physical shape, which only confused him. I asked what was going on in his life, and he shrugged. I looked at his chart and saw his birthday: he was going to turn forty in a week. I asked how he felt about that and out spilled one of the most gut-wrenching confessions of failure I have ever heard from a corporate vice-president. The man said he had even considered suicide rather than face up to his lack of accomplishment. He said that he had decided against suicide, yet I knew—and I told him—that if he did not reevaluate his vision of himself and his life, he would be committing a slow form of suicide. I remain very concerned about that patient; and at the time I found myself consumed by his dilemma because I have seen patients twice his age feel young and vibrant, excited about each new day.

You're as young as you feel is no longer just a banal cliche. It's a medical fact. You're also as young as you behave. Youthfulness is very much a state of mind, a mental outlook, an emotional feeling. There is a child within all of us all the time, whether we know it or not. When we are at our most stubborn, obstinate, and selfish we are allowing that child to be heard.

But we can also experience the positive emotions: the joy of discovery, the anticipation of what life has waiting for us. These youthful feelings never disappear. They are merely forgotten, along with thousands of other thoughts and emotions all stored away in the mind. Just as some of us forget how to add, subtract, divide, multiply, spell "precocious," or be nice to people, some of us just forget how to be young. Young is not a number. It is being active, feeling alive, vibrant, involved, and connected to the world—whether we are in the mood or not.

Growing younger, I believe, cannot happen to our bodies until it first begins to happen to our minds. Yet experience has led me to believe that the best way to change the mind is through moving the body, by doing, not by dreaming or rationalizing or any other cognitive act. By putting our bodies where our minds should be, our minds can soon catch up. How we live and how we die are, to a much greater degree than we have ever known before, functions of how we see ourselves, how we perceive reality. These factors can be choices.

MIND OVER IMMUNITY

As early as the second century A.D., when Greek philosopher-physician Galen observed that melancholic women tended to develop breast cancer much more often than their more jovial counterparts, there has been evidence linking the brain and the power of emotions to the effectiveness of the human immune system. History is full of plagues in which contagious diseases killed thousands, even millions; yet millions of other people exposed to the same potentially fatal disease somehow survived. Until recently, however, the medical establishment believed that immunity worked entirely as a separate entity from the brain.

The idea that we can, through our outlook on life, affect the way our body defends us against invading illness has received wide recognition only in the last five to seven years.

Recent studies have shown that stress reduces Natural Killer (NK) cells needed to kill invading germs and bacteria; another study showed stress to suppress lymphocytes, another immune system protector we rely on to defend against diseases such as cancer from inside and out. Most all of us have probably heard of at least one instance of a widow or widower mysteriously dying two weeks or so after losing her or his spouse. This is no longer a mystery. The will to live, or the lack of it, may prove to be more powerful than any drug. And the rest of the emotional gamut, it becomes clearer and clearer, has a profound effect on human health—probably more so than diet or even exercise.

HURRY UP DISEASE: THE #1 KILLER OF THE 1980s

For some it's a lifestyle—call it fast living; for others it is just an attitude of wanting "to get this over with," as if life itself is a tedium, a chore. Either way, the result is stress. Common symptoms are irritable bowel syndrome, constipation, frequent headaches, fatigue, chest and muscle pains, breathlessness, arthritis, skin disorders and itches, and, of course, ulcers.

There are perhaps as many different ways to become stressful as there are people. A patient of mine whose blood pressure had risen substantially from her previous visit gave me the following explanation: "It's all the driving I have to do." She had become a junior partner with a very big law firm in downtown Los Angeles, but she did not want to give up "the tranquility" of living near the beach, fifteen miles away. The hour commute was frustrating and terrifying. I suggested carpooling to work, which did not appeal to her. "To have to rely on someone picking me up to get to work? Too much anxiety." I suggested changing her hours to avoid the worst of the traffic, but in her new important position it was improper for her to arrive at the same time as the clerks and secretaries. I suggested alternative streets to take downtown, but they all seemed too complicated, which, of course, would cause more stress. I suggested she not pay attention to the traffic, then, but get some tapes of relaxing music and try to enjoy the ride. *No, relaxing music made her nervous.* It is amazing how creative—even amusing—some of us are when it comes to producing stress in our lives. The long-term price we pay for this stress, however, is not so creative or amusing. My patient the attorney eventually learned to relax after being hospitalized following a severe attack of hyperventilation.

Anger-induced high blood pressure is almost a proverb. But it is still worth emphasizing. I once had a forty-seven-year-old man come to my office complaining—and I mean *complaining*—of high blood pressure. He was the angriest man I had ever encountered. He did not wish to talk to me other than to say that he had been to five other doctors and none of them could cure his problem. I took his blood pressure and found it dangerously high, one of the highest I had seen in a man his age, and had an intuition about what was killing him. The man was so abrasive, however, I dared not inquire beyond the most superficial of questions about his condition. I gave him some blood pressure pills, told him to cut out alcohol and cigarettes, and put him on a salt-free diet and an exercise program. He went out and followed my advice compulsively—he even mapped out a sodium chart, an exercise schedule, a pill swallowing schedule—but his blood pressure did not come down. This made him more furious at the world and at me. His high blood pressure was now my fault, and it was rising to a new and extremely dangerous level. He screamed so violently that other patients could hear him and were growing frightened. Finally, I dared to confront the man. I told him he was drowning in a sea of anger; that he needed psychotherapy or at least a punching bag on which to let out his frustration, or he would die. Confrontation is not guaranteed to wake people up, but at that moment I felt it was his only hope. He stormed out of my office, threatening to sue me for malpractice. Within a month, however, my angry patient returned to my office, without the anger. He said that he had taken a long look at himself and saw the sheer insanity of his wrath: mad at the world, punishing only himself. He said he drove to Sears, bought three punching bags (one for home, one for his office, a small one for his car) and the next day called a therapist. He said to me, "Go ahead, Doc, take my blood pressure." I did. It was normal. "Those punching bags," he said, "they're better than your goddamn pills!"

He was right: all the medical knowledge and skill in the world cannot contend with the manifestations of the negative emotions. Other patients of mine who have had coronaries and are on the road to recovery still experience such fear right before I take their blood pressure—fear that their blood pressure will be high—that they cause the reading to be alarmingly high. I have to talk to them, calm them down, then get a more realistic reading. A recent study at University of California at San Francisco indicates that any of the negative moods and emotions can make blood pressure rise, including depression.

My experience with Hurry Up Disease, in my own life and in the lives of my patients, has led me to realize that there is an overriding dynamic: a need to control. We aim our anger and hostility at anyone or anything that might stand in the way of omnipotent control over life and surroundings. Fear, for many people, comes from the possibility they might lose some great deal of control, while hopelessness and depression can be created by the belief that control is forever lost, without the acceptance of this as part of the human condition. The truth is that none of us is in complete control of anything, and there is little if anything beyond the walls of our skin over which we have any lasting control. This realization can be to our advantage. It means that we can stop worrying about the world around us and begin to take responsibility for the emotions that are so closely linked to our health and longevity.

I have suggested to some of my patients several practical techniques for overcoming the need to control and have seen some positive results. I ask them to give up their anger by making a list of everything that makes them mad—from in-laws to neighbors, politics, traffic, even the smallest annoyance—and then follow up the angry laundry with an affirmation of joy and self-love. I have them write out their forgiveness to each person or thing (they don't have to send them to the person; just the act of forgiving is usually enough). Next I have them write out a list of all their perceived obligations and priorities. This list is interesting because it usually leaves out one particular priority: themselves. With a red pen I have them cross out all the so-called obligations that could, realistically, be left undone. This list of demands and pressures is often reduced by half—as is their high blood pressure and other symptoms. I have also prescribed meditation, hatha yoga, Gregorian chants, and cognitive therapy—all of which can work if you are truly willing to change.

LONELINESS IS A HEALTH ISSUE

Not long ago Dr. Harold Morowitz of Yale University looked at men who died premature deaths and grouped them according to marital status. He found that married men, smokers as well as nonsmokers, were half as likely to die as divorced and widowed men, and about 25 percent less likely to die than single men. Recent medical literature is full of other studies linking loneliness and alienation to illness and death, finding that people with a solid network of family and/or friends—even pets!—tend to be considerably more physically healthy in every way. This merely confirms to me what I have witnessed in my own medical practice for years.

Almost every day I see people who feel disenfranchised, unconnected, lonely, and isolated. Some live alone, while others may have a spouse and six children but still feel that way. Many of them are starved for human contact. They come to see me with minor ailments just so that someone will look at them, spend a little time caring for them, and touch them. Knowing that the degree to which we feel connected and vital to the world will very likely determine how well we are and how long we will live, I once again step out of the physician's limited role to encourage them to connect, with themselves and with others.

I have prescribed a variety of things to my many lonely patients. For some I suspect therapy might be in order; for most, joining a museum, a hiking group, a political movement, or volunteering at a hospital or soup kitchen can be tremendously beneficial. There are countless ways to escape loneliness by giving service to others—being a big brother or big sister, being a companion to another lonely person—or by being good to ourselves: getting a professional massage, for example, once or twice a week.

Just as emotions can directly affect our physical well being, so taking a concrete physical action that makes you more of a participant in the world can do wonders to relieve loneliness. I have seen it work with countless patients of mine, and I have used this philanthropic philosophy to deal with my own occasional feelings of loneliness. Of course, we must consider our own feelings; we must be aware of them and realize their importance, but ultimately we are probably more likely to change our feelings not by thinking about them but by getting out in the world and participating in something.

For many of us this can mean having to reconsider some of our values, perhaps less for the good of humankind than for the good of our own health.

THE MORE-THAN-7% SOLUTION

Whenever I encounter a patient I believe might be suffering the manifestations of an emotional syndrome I will often pose the question: "What do you consider your most important needs in life?"

The answers are often predictable: food, money, sex, (sometimes but not often) love. I rarely hear about creative needs, the need to feel useful, the need for music, poetry, art, or the need to watch the sky turn yellow, orange, purple, then dark. Yet these are all very basic human necessities. Part of rising above loneliness, despair, anger, or stress, I have discovered, is a realization of what one's needs are, and a commitment to satisfying them.

All of us must somehow function in a world of mortgage or rent payments, insurance premiums, job markets, corporate politics, freeway traffic, and noise pollution; but it is possible to live healthfully—mentally and physically—in this world, provided we remain in touch with the rest of the earth. I'm not saying we must trade in our business clothes for a loincloth and pitch a permanent tent, or that we have to join the Sierra Club, or even go camping. But each of us is going to be a lot saner, a lot healthier, and probably live longer if we regularly find some time in our lives to hug a tree (at least figuratively) and commune with a rock.

Good health, I firmly believe, depends upon perspective. We must maintain a strong sense of who we are and what life really means to us. This means owning material things without allowing them to own us. Our security, material or otherwise, comes from some kind of faith in ourselves, in the world, and, if we are comfortable with it, a spiritual belief.

Many people easily grasp all the principles I am now suggesting (none of which has originated with me) once they have had a close encounter with death—once they have recovered from the first heart attack or learned that they have cancer or any other illness which reminds them of their inevitable mortality. Some people believe they really cannot fully appreciate life until they have had a close call. I disagree. There is no need to wait. We can all start taking better care of ourselves emotionally while we are as healthy as we can possibly be.

Since I am not a trained expert in the field of mental health, I do not expect all of my patients, or all of my readers, to consider my advice the final word. Not by any means. I believe the answers lie within us all, provided we are willing to look. The most I can hope for in these pages is to convince you of how important the body-mind connection is and how much our attitudes affect our health. This means that the next time you go to a restaurant and order *unbuttered* salmon but it comes with butter all over it and there is no time to send it back, you should remember that butter is less crucial to your health than the anger you may put yourself through. In that situation my advice is: Relax and eat the butter. And the next time some unforeseen crisis prevents you from exercising, remember: the anger and worry you may choose to subject yourself to will do far more damage than missing one day's exercise.

Finally, perhaps the greatest advice I can remind you of is something I tell my radio listeners every week. Don't forget to take, and to give, lots of vitamin L: that's *love.* We need to fill our lives with people we love, and we have to learn to love ourselves, unconditionally, no matter what fools we make of ourselves in the world. Without a daily dosage of vitamin L, no one's prescription for longevity is complete.

Part Two

Rejuvenation Plans for Specific Symptoms and Ailments

At this point you are well on your way to living well into the twenty-first century, to helping your physician give you the best kind of care available, and to making your life insurance agent a very happy person. But for those who already suffer from chronic conditions, the specific plans in this section build on the basic Rejuvenation Diet and program in order to maximize your assault on these illnesses.

For some of you, rejuvenation and longevity may depend on becoming aware of an addiction: to alcohol, to cigarettes, to over-the-counter as well as prescription medications, or even certain foods. Addictions, whether they are obvious to us or not, are a major obstruction to the kind of nutrition and lifestyle that promotes long-term good health. If not dealt with they can negate all of our best efforts with our Rejuvenation Diet and with our supplemental plans. But we do not have to have them—not from now on.

For others of you, allergies may pose a similar barrier, and so they too will be dealt with in this section, both to give you an awareness of what they are and what are some of the most common kinds, along with some general guidelines and tips for those of you to whom it applies, so that they will not stand in the way of anyone's longevity and good health.

Then follow the plans, which present the most current and exciting and effective means for you (under the supervision of a responsible physician) to identify and overcome the following common ailments: anemia, arthritis, asthma, bronchitis, cancer, constipation, depression, diabetes, diverticulitis, emphysema, Epstein-Barr virus (a recent epidemic), fibrocystic breast disease, chronic headaches, heart disease, herpes, high cholesterol, high blood pressure, hyperthyroidism, hypothyroidism, indigestion, irritable bowel syndrome, kidney stones, lower back pain, malabsorption syndrome, obesity, osteoporosis, chronic pain, psoriasis, stress, transient ischemic attack, ulcers, urinary tract infections, and vision problems.

Some of these ailments are illnesses, others are symptoms of illnesses; all are formidable obstacles to good health, comfort, joy, and longevity. Each condition will be defined along with an explanation of possible causes and usual symptoms, followed by some general information that may help you to help your doctor give effective treatment, as well as nutritional guidelines to alleviate and improve the condition. In most all of the plans this means emphasizing certain rejuvenation foods and increasing certain supplemental insurance; in some plans we may need to avoid certain rejuvenation foods, at least temporarily. Where applicable, I will address the issues of exercise and lifestyle, though for many of these ailments, if you've begun to implement the suggestions in Chapters 5 and 6 you may already be feeling their positive effects.

If you currently suffer from more than one of these conditions, you may have to make a choice as to which specific diet and plan to follow first. While most of them are compatible with one another, there are exceptions. Yams, for example, are wonderful if your problem is diverticulitis or high cholesterol, but they must be limited if you are diabetic. Some of us must therefore set up priorities, deciding what is our most pressing health problem. I give my own patients the following criteria:

NUMBER ONE PRIORITY

Any serious condition which, if not altered, may lead to serious health complications. These include high cholesterol, high blood pressure, and transient ischemic attacks.

SECOND PRIORITY

Any condition that prevents good digestion. Without proper digestion, much of what we eat will be of little use to us.

AFTER THAT

Any other condition which stands in the way of good health, quality of life, and longevity.

Some people need as few as three weeks to become symptom-free or to bring a chronic disease under control. For others, six to nine months may be in order. For those with substance addictions, a day-to-day commitment over a lifetime will reap its rewards in good health and longevity. Some of you may find following some of my recommendations to be a conscious effort—at least for a while. They should not, however, become arduous; relax and enjoy them. Living longer better is not a matter of guilt or unproductive anxiety about our current condition.

Ailments are not some form of cosmic punishment, or even self-punishment. Every illness is an opportunity to become a better, healthier person. It is a chance to grow.

Addiction Plan

IDENTIFICATION AND CAUSES

A vast number of different substance addictions may prevent anyone from obtaining optimum health, growing younger, and, in fact, having much hope of longevity. Undealt-with addictions will, in fact, age us prematurely. These addictions can be of three kinds: alcohol, drug (including cigarettes), or food.

There are many ways to define an addiction. The most profound, in my opinion, comes from an ancient Chinese description of alcoholism, translated to mean: "A man takes a drink, a drink takes a drink, and then the drink takes the man." In medicine we view an addiction as a dependency on a substance (or behavior) such that the cessation of the substance (or behavior) causes severe trauma: withdrawal symptoms and disabilities.

Substance abuse can cause brain deterioration, severe nutritional deficiencies, and muscular weakness. Alcoholism in particular can cause liver disease, cirrhosis, gastrointestinal disease, impotence, ulcers, bleeding disorders, heart disease, and, it has been recently proven, cancer. The side effects of drug addictions range anywhere from mild depression to suicide—and include the 1 in 600 people who die every year from long-term addiction to cigarettes—while compulsive overeating invariably leads to obesity, which leads to years of suffering and disability and a shortened life-span. But perhaps equally serious, some of these addictions can cause loss of family, friends, productivity, and income. We all deserve better for ourselves.

SYMPTOMS

To know whether you are an alcoholic, a drug addict, or a compulsive overeater requires honesty and courage. There are many books on the subject, some of which I will recommend in the appendix, but none of which can effect any change if a person will not take a truthful look into the mirror. Alcoholics Anonymous puts out a questionnaire with which to determine if a person has a drinking problem. Narcotics Anonymous and Overeaters Anonymous have adopted their own twenty questions. These can be obtained at any local AA, NA, or OA office. But as far as I'm concerned, here's a foolproof test.

Consider again what I have outlined as the healthy approach to living: no more than my recommended amounts of alcohol per day, the complete elimination of illegal narcotics, cigarettes, and caffeine, no more habitual use and misuse of over-the-counter medicines, a serious reevaluation (with your physician) of the need for tranquilizers, along with a low-fat, low-calorie, high-fiber diet (without diet pills!). While many of us may be set in our ways, resistant to change, and lazy, if the desire is there, change will take place. If desire is there yet you find it physically impossible to implement these life-enhancing measures, then it may well be likely you have an addiction to one or more substances.

TREATMENT

If you are addicted, I urge you to begin a program of complete abstinence and to seek out moral, psychological, and spiritual support. Alcoholics Anonymous has a very impressive record, as do the other Anonymous programs: Narcotics Anonymous, Overeaters Anonymous, Smokers Anonymous. They succeed, I have learned, because they show the addict that he or she is not alone and that others have overcome the same addiction. According to these programs, such addictions are never "cured" but can be arrested through complete abstinence from the destructive substance or the destructive behavior—one day at a time—and through dealing with the underlying causes of addiction: the thoughts and feelings that instigated the need for sedation. The right therapist can offer much-needed additional support.

For cigarette smoking, the best program is to decide that you don't want to die a horrid, suffocating death, and to quit cold turkey, surrounding yourself with people who love you no matter how irritable you temporarily become. The American Lung Association and the Seventh Day Adventists also have successful programs for quitting smoking.

Once the addiction cycle has been broken there is no longer any reason for it to compromise health or shorten life. But since there are possible withdrawal symptoms to confront, and potential physical damage to be repaired, I will recommend the most up-to-date nutritional guidelines for easing the discomfort of withdrawal and for rebuilding our bodies.

I cannot emphasize enough, however, that diet and supplements are only one part of the recovery equation: without exercise and a healthy outlook on life, you will nourish yourself to no avail. The most important prescription with which to challenge any addiction is a belief in yourself.

EASING WITHDRAWALS

In helping recovering addicts in my own practice, I have discovered some very useful nutritional tips for easing physical withdrawals—provided that a rigorous program is already in place dealing with the mental and emotional aspects of the addiction. Mangos have been found to contain a natural antidepressant chemical for many people, which science is not yet able to explain, and one mango a day can help to relieve some withdrawal symptoms. I also recommend home-cooked, unbuttered, unsalted popcorn for those who find they need constant oral satisfaction. The following supplementation plan should accompany the standard rejuvenation supplementation insurance prescribed in Chapter 3.

SUPPLEMENTS INCREASED FROM REGULAR REJUVENATION INSURANCE

L-tryptophan	500 mgs, four times a day, along with:
B-6	10 to 25 mgs daily
B-complex	50 mgs, twice a day
Vitamin C	500 mgs, four to six times a day
L-glutamine	500 mgs twice a day

REBUILDING THE BODY

The most important part of your recovery is clearly your emotional state. Once your psychological balance begins to return, the body can begin to rebuild.

Our Rejuvenation Diet by itself will help our bodies to rebuild themselves during recovery from most drug addictions, including cigarette smoking and caffeine. Once we are free of the drug, our bodies can absorb and use all the nutrients we take in and the rejuvenation process can begin to happen. I urge you, however, to have a complete medical examination to determine if you are dangerously deficient in any specific nutrient. For a sustained overeating disorder, you may want to consider the additional measures suggested in the Obesity Plan, to follow.

Regarding recovery from alcoholism I can suggest some universal nutritional techniques to help expedite the rebuilding process. Although excess alcohol generally causes similar nutritional deficiencies, everyone is unique, and so I advise a complete medical examination before undergoing the following program.

If you are recovering from alcoholism, you probably will have a strong craving for sugar; excess alcohol consumption seems to deplete the brain's supply of the neurotransmitter serotonin. This deficiency can cause anxiety, irritability, and depression. Sugar temporarily raises serotonin levels, relieving these symptoms. Refined sugars do this the fastest, and so they are most often craved, but refined sugars also produce an insulin response, creating a physical and psychological depression that can be worse than the one you are trying to relieve. Hence the first order of business is to make sure we get our sugar from *complex* carbohydrates. Fresh fruits, lots of them, are a crucial part of the recovering alcoholics diet. They relieve the craving for sweets and give us high levels of nutrients and good fiber. Eat them liberally at first. Once you're past the withdrawal phase, I still recommend the antidepressant mango. Other important fruits are papayas, kiwis, bananas, cantaloupes, oranges, grapes, and berries; they are high in minerals, especially potassium and magnesium, which most alcoholics are dangerously deficient in, and they are also high in natural sugar that is released slowly in the body.

Since many alcoholics are severely malnourished, I relax the limit on fresh fruits from three to five per day, provided it is accompanied with a protein source (about one ounce of protein per fruit). We want to maintain a solid balance between complex carbohydrates—fresh fruit, fresh vegetables, and whole grains—and good low-fat protein sources such as fish, white meat chicken, tofu, nonfat yogurt, cheese, and other nonfat dairy products. The rebuilding body needs a higher percentage of protein, and carbohydrates boost the rebuilding power of the amino acids while protein slows the release of sugar from complex carbohydrates in the body. Eating every three to four hours is not a bad idea, and I should reemphasize that ten to fourteen glasses a day of clean filtered water is crucial.

The newly recovering alcoholic has specific vitamin, mineral, and amino acid insurance needs to help maintain normal serotonin levels and to rapidly replace the B vitamins in which most alcoholics are so deficient.

SUPPLEMENTS INCREASED FROM REGULAR REJUVENATION LEVELS

L-tryptophan	500 mgs, four times a day
Niacin	25 mgs with each dose of L-tryptophan
B-6	25 mgs with each dose of L-tryptophan
B-complex	100 to 150 mgs daily

THE EXERCISE FACTOR

A good long walk can stop hyperventilation and other symptoms of anxiety produced by withdrawals, and should be a part of your anti-addiction program. See Chapter 5.

LIFESTYLE CONSIDERATIONS

Meditation and yoga also work on the psychological traumas that accompany the breaking of bad habits. See Chapter 6.

Allergy Plan

IDENTIFICATION AND CAUSES

An allergy is a response by the body to a substance that is viewed as an unfriendly invader. There are many substances we ingest that can cause a vast barrage of uncomfortable and potentially dangerous effects. Any food that causes an allergic reaction in us, whether it's anti-rejuvenating chocolate or "health-promoting" broccoli, should be considered personally "toxic" by definition. Any allergy left untreated can block the effectiveness of our Rejuvenation Diet and any other diet in any of the subsequent plans, since, among other things, it can cause our immune system to attack rather than defend us.

SYMPTOMS

The body sets off a variety of chemical defense mechanisms, manifesting in sneezes, runny nose and eyes, itches, mood swings, anxiety attacks, depression, hyperactivity, bad dreams, hallucinations, vertigo, headaches, and almost any other horrific symptom one can imagine. Allergies can even mimic other illnesses such as viral infections, common colds, stomach aches, peptic ulcers, respiratory infections, and arthritis.

TREATMENT

There is a new breed of doctor, now, the clinical ecologist, who treats these kinds of allergy-provoking symptoms. Yet it may still be up to you, if you are having unexplained symptoms, to suggest the possibility of an allergy to your general physician to help him help you. When I was a student, for example, we were told that the substances likely to cause allergic reactions were chocolates, nuts, dairy products, citrus, eggs, feathers, cotton, dog and cat hairs, and pollen. Now we know that any food or any food additive can potentially cause an allergic reaction in someone. Several recent studies concluded that celery eaten one hour before exercising can cause volatile allergic reactions in some people. Estimates of human illness caused by food allergies range as high as 60 percent. This means that part of taking care of ourselves is finding out what foods do not agree with us and eliminating them from our lives.

It is my firm belief that many of us may be allergic to refined sugars and refined carbohydrates, to saturated and polyunsaturated fats, to caffeine and cigarettes, and to any or all of the thousands of chemical additives and pesticides that have invaded our food supply. By eliminating or cutting down drastically on these toxins as recommended in the Rejuvenation Diet, we will have already cut out some serious threats to our health, and many of you will notice the extinction of a variety of unpleasant symptoms that you may have thought were chronic conditions, an inevitable part of life. But there are certain foods considered good for most people, from fruits and vegetables to grains and nonfat dairy—even vitamin pills, if they are not "hypoallergenic"—which may provoke allergic reactions in some of you.

A mental state of optimism and calm may help diminish the allergy, but it will not make it go away. Nor will age. It is a myth that we outgrow all of our allergies. Moreover, exercise can actually temporarily increase the likelihood and intensity of an allergic reaction, as was recently discovered with joggers who ate celery one hour before running. This does not mean, please, that we should ever consider compromising our exercise program. What it does mean is that it is possible that something as seemingly benign as a green bean might cause a headache, dizziness, irritable bowels, or any of countless other physical and mental symptoms. Keep exercising. If you're allergic to green beans or to celery, stop eating them.

If you think you might have a food allergy, the first step you need to take is to have an allergy workup by your physician or an allergist. It may be possible, through keeping a food diary, to identify a food allergy yourself; but this is risky. It may, after all, not be a food allergy; allergies can be caused by skin contact and inhalation as well as by food. A medical professional is probably needed to remedy the problem, but you can certainly help by keeping a close awareness of the foods you eat and your body's reaction, and by detoxifying your home as much as possible. Once the allergy is identified, and if it is a food allergy, it shouldn't be hard to find an equally nutritious and delicious substitute for the culprit food.

The books listed in the Recommended Reading section of this book can help you and your doctor identify food allergies and avoid allergy-causing foods and substances so that you may get on with more enjoyable things in life.

Anemia Plan

IDENTIFICATION AND CAUSES

Anemia is a quantitative deficiency of the body's red blood cells, which are vital to carrying oxygen throughout the body. It is most commonly caused by a deficiency of iron in the diet or by a problem in absorbing or metabolizing iron because of drug use or other factors. Other causes are internal bleeding, such as ulcers, bleeding intestines, or chronically bleeding stomach irritated by the excessive use of aspirin and/or anti-inflammatory drugs, and external bleeding from female menstrual flow or blood lost from hemorrhoids or cancers. Anemia can also be caused by a deficiency in vitamins B-6, B-12, folic acid, and vitamin C, either from inadequate vitamin intake or a failure to properly absorb these crucial vitamins. Some anemias, such as thalassemia major and minor, and hemolytic anemia (common among those of Mediterranean decent) are hereditary, but anemia may just as likely be a reaction to birth control, or even, as recent evidence has found, jogging regularly on pavement, which can destroy red blood cells. Anemia can also be a symptom of certain cancers, tumors, polyps (benign or malignant), or hypothyroidism, and thus must be taken seriously and treated under the guidance of your physician.

SYMPTOMS

Anemia can cause a variety of unpleasant symptoms. Most common are fatigue, tiredness, chilliness, poor memory, and depression. Other frequent symptoms are shortness of breath with heart palpitations, recurring vertigo, anxiety and tension, easy bruising, and a diminished libido. Advanced anemias can cause severe pallor as well as pale and brittle finger and toenails.

TREATMENT

If any of these symptoms are present for more than two weeks, a serum ferritin (blood iron) analysis is absolutely necessary. This will not only determine whether or not you are suffering from anemia but it will also establish whether there is an iron deficiency even if red blood cell count is normal. Recent evidence has proven that some people suffer the symptoms of anemia without diminished red blood cell count, and an uninformed physician, if he or she has not checked serum ferritin levels, can make a misdiagnosis and fail to treat the problem correctly. Once your physician has identified the presence of an anemia, the cause is clear and treatment will likely include an iron or B-12 supplement, taken orally, or, if the cause of the anemia is an absorption problem, the vitamin or mineral may have to be given as an injection, or intestinal therapy may be indicated.

ANTI-ANEMIA DIET

Hereditary anemias, such as thalassemia major and minor, and hemolytic are not diet-related, hence there is nothing in these pages that I can prescribe other than a competent physician or hematologist. In cases of iron deficiency anemia and pernicious anemia (caused by lack of B-12 and/or folic acid absorption), the dietary measures I commonly prescribe to my patients can help you in your treatment. Once I have diagnosed these anemias (or low iron levels without the anemia) and begun to address any physiological causes, I steer the patient in the direction of a high-iron or high–B-12 or high–folic acid diet. Since we want to stay away from red meat, whose high iron content comes at a high-cholesterol, high-fat price, the anti-anemia diet is built around nonfat dairy, high-iron complex carbohydrates, fish, poultry, and only the leanest meat.

REJUVENATION FOODS TO EMPHASIZE FOR IRON DEFICIENCY ANEMIA

Dairy

Yogurt, nonfat cheese, nonfat milk.

Vegetables

Cabbage, green vegetables (especially turnip greens, asparagus, broccoli, parsley, watercress), beets, carrots, baked yams, and potatoes (especially the skins).

Whole grains

Wheat germ and brown rice.

Fruits

Black cherries (and their juice), dried apricots,* raisins,* bananas.

Other good iron sources

Sunflower seeds, black beans, amazaki drink (a delicious Japanese soy beverage found in health food stores and Japanese markets).

FOR PERNICIOUS (POOR B-12 ABSORPTION) ANEMIA

All fish and poultry, nonfat yogurt, nonfat milk, nonfat cheese, beans, green vegetables, whole grains.

SUPPLEMENTS INCREASED FROM REGULAR REJUVENATION INSURANCE

If your doctor discovers an iron deficiency anemia and prescribes an iron supplement tablet, you will want to take the iron supplement with dinner (unless your doctor indicates otherwise), and you can help the absorption of the iron with 1000 extra milligrams of vitamin C. Avoid alcohol, coffee, tea, or anything containing caffeine or tanic acid, and avoid stress; these things will interfere with the badly needed iron. And make sure your doctor keeps a close watch on your serum ferritin level so that excess iron intake does not continue longer than necessary. Injections of B-12 are needed for pernicious anemia.

THE EXERCISE FACTOR

A regular exercise program as prescribed in Chapter 5 will help with general health, which can only help to speed up recovery. Jogging may not be advisable, but walking will; make sure to get a pair of comfortable, well-padded walking shoes.

---

*Dried apricots and raisins are preferred over regular apricots and grapes because the dried fruit is more concentrated in iron and you therefore do not need to eat as much.

LIFESTYLE CONSIDERATIONS

Chapter 6 says it all.

Arthritis Plan

IDENTIFICATION AND CAUSES

There are somewhere in the neighborhood of 120 different diseases that fall into the category known as arthritis. What they all have in common is inflammation and pain of the joints, a very debilitating affliction. I will not attempt to cover all 120 in these pages but will deal with the most common forms and recommend some good books for further in-depth reading.

There are three very general types of arthritis that we can identify. Noninflammatory arthritis, such as osteoarthritis, is caused by the degeneration of cartilage at the edge of bones from wear and tear, degeneration from abuse, or trauma, such as an injury. Inflammatory arthritis, currently the most common type, afflicts bones, muscles, tendons, or connective tissue; it can be caused by autoimmune chemicals that destroy membranes and linings of the bones, as in the case of rheumatoid arthritis, or by stress, or may even be the result of a food allergy. The third general category of arthritis is infectious arthritis, caused by any number of viral or bacterial infections in the joints. Other causes of arthritis include hyperthyroidism and gout, an excess of uric acid in the blood which can bring on a gouty arthritis. In all cases of arthritis, alcohol, coffee, excess salt and refined sugar, and cigarettes will most often exacerbate the condition, as will tension, anger, and other negative emotions.

SYMPTOMS

The most common symptom of all forms of arthritis is pain in one or in many joints and bones. But arthritis can also cause fevers, headaches, redness and tenderness of joints, muscle aches, and a general sense of illness. In the case of rheumatoid arthritis, which is a general system illness, there may be fever, weight loss, morning stiffness, and a general malaise; rest almost always lessens the symptoms, whereas stress and fatigue almost always make them worse.

TREATMENT

There are many drugs used in the treatment of arthritis, aspirin still being the most widely used and least supervised. Other medications commonly used are nonsteroidal anti-inflammatory drugs. These block certain body chemicals called prostaglandins, which cause arthritic pain. But many arthritis medicines take effect slowly, and many of them have undesirable side effects, some of which have been known to be worse than the arthritis itself (see The Nutrition-Drug Connection, Chapter 4). I am always very careful in prescribing medications to patients suffering from arthritis. Please make sure your doctor considers all of your alternatives.

The latest breakthrough, so new your physician may not even have heard of it yet, regards *Substance-P,* and it is, in fact, still unknown to many physicians, even those studying in the field of rheumatology. Substance-P is a chemical discharged from the spinal cord nerves when we are under great emotional stress. Studies have found that Substance-P stimulates the cells of the linings of joints to release inflammatory prostaglandins. This brings on joint inflammation and swelling attacks in those people with rheumatoid arthritis. Ask your doctor to find out about this important discovery.

Also very important: make sure your doctor checks your kidneys; while arthritis can be caused by kidney trouble, it may also instigate kidney trouble. Since arthritis can be caused by a food allergy, an allergy workup is essential in prescribing treatment.

Arthritis no longer need be a hopeless condition. Through diet, exercise, and lifestyle changes we can do much to alleviate this brutal ailment.

ANTI-ARTHRITIS DIET

The guidelines of the Rejuvenation Diet will help enormously in both prevention and treatment of all forms of arthritis, but within the realm of whole natural foods there are some foods we want to be careful with and others we want to emphasize. Citrus fruits and juices may exacerbate an arthritic condition, as can high concentrations of refined sugars. The foods we want to focus on are fresh fish containing EPA omega-3 (listed below) and olive oil, both of which have recently been linked to a diminishing of certain arthritic conditions in some people. We want to eat vegetables, fruits, and grains, all high in vitamin and mineral concentration, and nonfat dairy products that will not produce allergic reactions. (For many people, goat cheese and nonfat yogurt are safe alternatives to other dairy products.) We also want to make an extra effort to drink *at least* twelve glasses of fresh, filtered water per day.

REJUVENATION FOODS TO EMPHASIZE

Vegetables

Alfalfa sprouts (or tablets), cabbage, carrots, cauliflower, garlic, kale, kohlrabi, parsley, soy products (such as tofu).

Fruits (limit to three per day)

Apples, avocados, bananas, cherries, mangoes, papayas.

Whole grains

Oatmeal, rolled oats, oat bran, brown rice, wheat germ.

Dairy

Goat cheese and nonfat yogurt.

EPA omega-3 fish

Salmon, tuna, sardines, halibut, mackerel, herring, squid, shark.

SUPPLEMENTS INCREASED FROM REGULAR REJUVENATION INSURANCE

Niacinamide*	200 to 300 mgs, twice a day
Pantothenic acid*	500 mgs, twice a day
B-6	25 mgs
Vitamin E	400 IUs daily
Calcium	1500 mgs daily
Magnesium	100 mgs daily
Manganese	50 mgs daily
Chelated potassium	99 mgs, two tablets daily
Selenium	50 mcgs, twice a day
Chelated chromium	100 mcgs daily
Zinc (picolinate)	30 mgs daily
L-tryptophan	500 mgs, four times a day, taken on empty stomach
EPA omega-3**	four capsules, two after lunch, two after dinner
Wheat bran	six tablets daily

THE EXERCISE FACTOR

Exercise is crucial to the treatment of arthritis and the management of its pain. Despite previous beliefs that exercise worsened the arthritic condition, we now know the opposite is true. I have seen countless patients drastically reduce arthritic pain

*I have seen joint mobility increased with these excessive doses of niacinamide and pantothenic acid; however these substances in such quantities may upset the stomach, in which case you should try half the dosage or if necessary, return to regular rejuvenation daily dosage.

**Be sure when selecting an EPA omega-3 supplement to choose one that is pure. There are some on the market that contain other substances, potentially toxic. The use of the capsules in place of eating fish is still controversial and not necessarily conclusive or founded; four to six ounces of salmon equals three EPA capsules. Do not use if you are taking aspirin.

by walking. Hatha yoga can be very helpful, as it relieves physical and emotional stress, further diminishing pain, while avoiding overextention. Exercising the arms, legs, and other joints in warm water or a hot tub has become popular with some of my patients. Being in water reduces gravity, making movement easier, and the relaxation is invaluable. I do, however, warn my patients not to stay too long in hot tubs or jacuzzis, and not to use them at all if they have high blood pressure, heart disease, vascular disease, or if they are taking muscle relaxants or analgesics.

LIFESTYLE CONSIDERATIONS

Since stress, anger, and other negative emotions aggravate arthritis and its ensuing pain, we obviously want to take a good hard look at the way we are choosing to live our lives. Realizing that our lifestyle and attitudes might be the direct cause of pain and deterioration, we must begin to balance the benefits of our belief systems and behaviors versus the shortcomings they produce. For some of us this means not looking up at the heavens and asking, "Why me?", but looking straight into the mirror, and asking, "Why are you doing this to me?" And consider yourself lucky. If arthritis causes you to give up your stress and anger, it may very well have saved you from a more fatal illness. Biofeedback and meditation can do wonders to relieve the pain, and sometimes helps to reverse the illness.

Asthma Plan

IDENTIFICATION AND CAUSES

There are two kinds of asthma, both characterized by a difficulty in exhaling. They differ primarily in cause. Intrinsic asthma is a marker of the presence of a lung disease, such as chronic obstructive pulmonary disease (see Emphysema Plan), or may be brought on by emotional stress, while extrinsic asthma is that which is not associated with another lung disorder and is usually precipitated by an allergic exposure, usually airborn pollen, mold, house dust, or animal dander.

SYMPTOMS

Shortness of breath, often accompanied by chest tightness or congestion, wheezing, and coughing are the most common symptoms of both kinds of asthma. If you experience them often for long periods of time, bring them to the attention of your doctor.

TREATMENT

Medical treatment often involves drugs such as cortisone or chromolyn sodium, a capsule placed in an inhaler and inhaled every six hours as a preventive measure to ward off asthmatic attack. Your doctor may also want to prescribe bronchial dilators such as theophylline, metaproterenol, or an aminophylline-derived drug, all of which should be carefully monitored and nutritionally accounted for (see The Nutrition-Drug Connection, Chapter 4). Allergy tests, pulmonary function tests, X rays, and other tests should be done to determine the cause and the best possible treatment. Often the only successful treatment is the avoidance of an allergenic substance, food, or inhalant, or appropriate measures to treat an existing lung disease. But there is one dietary factor, newly discovered, which may help, along with some lifestyle considerations.

ANTI-ASTHMA DIET

While the Rejuvenation Diet removes many potential allergenic foods from your daily consumption and assures adequate immune-stabilizing nutrients, two major studies have found a severe deficiency of vitamin B-6 in asthmatics. While it is in no way a cure or even a total treatment for asthma, testing to date confirms that elevated amounts of B-6 intake can decrease the occurrence, duration, and intensity of attacks in the asthmatics studied. Another current finding—so new that as I write this it has yet to be officially released—is the role of magnesium in the onset and treatment of asthma. To quote the study, published in the *Journal of the American Medical Association*, "Lower magnesium uptake or a deficiency of this mineral may play a role in some types of asthma, and may therefore be useful as a supplementary therapy in controlling bronchial asthma."

REJUVENATION FOODS TO EMPHASIZE

Vitamin B-6 sources

Fish, whole grains, beans, nonfat dairy, avocados, bananas.

Magnesium sources

Whole grains, green vegetables, celery,* bananas, pineapples, most beans.

SUPPLEMENTS INCREASED FROM REGULAR REJUVENATION INSURANCE

Vitamin B-6	100 mgs daily, along with your B-complex
Magnesium	500 mgs in the morning, 500 mgs in the evening

LIFESTYLE CONSIDERATIONS

Kiss your cigarettes good-bye and thank yourself for lengthening your life (and the lives of those close to you who share your air) by decades. You may have to do without certain types of fabric in your wardrobe, and—at the risk of sounding barbaric—pets may have to find new homes. Stress, as almost always, is a potential factor. See the Stress Plan.

Bronchitis Plan

IDENTIFICATION AND CAUSES

Bronchitis is an infection within the bronchial tubes of the lungs. These lead air to the outer reaches of the lung. It may be caused by acute infections, fever, and coughs, or it may be associated with other lung diseases. Most often it is brought on—and is always exacerbated—by smoking. Alcohol abuse,

*Never eat celery within an hour before exercising.

lack of exercise, stress, and poor sleeping habits may also be contributory factors. Allergies from food ingestion and inhalents can be causes, and should always be considered.

SYMPTOMS

A chronic cough containing sputum is a cause for concern and should be checked immediately to determine whether it is an indication of the presence of bronchitis.

TREATMENT

Respiratory therapy under the supervision of a physician is usually in order for the treatment of bronchitis, and if the condition is very severe, sometimes the lungs need to be washed out. In most cases, however, a heavy intake of fluids along with adequate rest, relaxation, and the discontinuation of exposure to any allergy-provoking substances—in food, air, clothes, or anywhere else—can do wonders and should be a part of any doctor's prescription for bronchitis. Sometimes antibiotics are needed, but always ask your doctor if they are absolutely essential, and make sure the prescription covers you only for as long as you need them, as antibiotics over long periods of time can compromise the immune system, making us more susceptible to recurring infection.

ANTI-BRONCHITIS DIET

The foods we want to concentrate on here are those that can help liquefy mucus secretion.

REJUVENATION FOODS TO EMPHASIZE

Fruits

Apricots, berries, oranges, grapefruits, mangoes, papayas, pineapples, kiwis, cantaloupes, watermelons, and any and all fruit juices (without added sugar).

Vegetables

Broccoli, Brussels sprouts, carrots, garlic, onions, dark green leafy vegetables, spinach, yams, steamed seaweed, any and all vegetable juices (without added salt), and any and all low—and I mean *very low*—sodium vegetable soups, preferably homemade.

Others

Chicken soup,* seafood, commercial herbal teas, nonfat milk, *and lots and lots of pure clean filtered water!*

SUPPLEMENTS INCREASED FROM REGULAR REJUVENATION INSURANCE

Beta carotene	25,000 IUs daily
Vitamin C**	1000 mgs, ten times a day *maximum*, or to tolerance
Garlic capsules**	as tolerated (Kyolic brand liquid)

THE EXERCISE FACTOR

Daily exercise, such as walking, is crucial for the recovery of bronchitis and other respiratory conditions, but there are other specific exercises that may also help. Respiratory exercises should be prescribed by a pulmonary therapist. One very simple exercise I have patients of mine perform is to blow bubbles into a glass of water through a straw. Another one is to blow out a candle, relighting and blowing for a sustained period of time. Hatha yoga training can teach countless breathing exercises, which I have seen help in the reduction of bronchitis obstruction and the accompanying wheezing in some of the most severe bronchitis cases I have encountered.

LIFESTYLE CONSIDERATIONS

For anyone with bronchitis, cigarette smoking is no longer merely unadvisable, it is a life-and-death ultimatum. But stress

*Watch out for excess sodium and for sulfites and nitrites in all commercial soups; better to make your own.

**If diarrhea occurs, decrease dosage until it subsides.

and anxiety must also be considered and dealt with (see the Stress Plan). We must be honest and take responsibility for how much of the condition we have either brought on or made worse.

Since the environmental hazards of certain working and living conditions can be major factors, we must have enough self-esteem to demand that we live and work without exposure to air that is making us sick. For some of us this may mean changing where we live and/or work, but there are also measures we can take to alleviate toxic exposure without altogether fleeing the scene. Many such tips are available in any number of good books, which I will recommend in the Recommended Reading section.

Cancer Plan

IDENTIFICATION AND CAUSES

Perhaps the word most feared in any doctor's office, *cancer*, refers to destructive cells which can occur in any part of the body. These cells do not respond to the basic law and order of the body but grow and overgrow into a premature different form of cell, reproducing at excessive rates, stealing all the necessary nutrients meant for normal cells, and causing depletion of all nutrients. Cancer cells can migrate all over the body, invading other tissues and growing abnormally, compressing and killing nearby normal cells. Early detection is therefore critical.

There are many different types of cancer, and many potential causes. All of us have some cancer cells forming in our body, though if our immunity is strong we are constantly fighting them off and never know it. Other cancers can invade our body through a variety of sources. It is well established that cancer occurs far more often in people who smoke, drink excessive alcohol, eat a lot of burned protein, and regularly consume high-fat high-caloric diets. New evidence links chewing tobacco not only to cancers in the mouth but also with a higher risk of kidney cancer. Also linked directly to kidney cancer is obesity. And some of the most recent findings have shown that deficiencies in selenium, vitamin B-6, and vitamin E severely increase the risk of many different kinds of cancers.

Cancer has also been associated with a myriad of environmental chemicals, including formaldehyde, which is used in artificial fiber carpets, plastics, cosmetics, and many other domestic substances. Saccharin sweetener has long been thought to cause cancer, as have many other artificial flavors, colors, and preservatives in foods. Free radicals, which are broken bits of molecules missing an electron and also the by-products of certain chemicals we are exposed to, increase aging and are known to induce cancer. Direct sunlight and possibly excess exposure to fluorescent lighting can, over time, develop malignant melanomas (skin cancer). The most recent data on cancer causation also points to certain viral infections. Papilloma virus and herpes virus, for example, can bring on some forms of cervical cancer in women. Kaposi sarcoma, occurring commonly (though not exclusively) in AIDS victims, is another virus associated with cancer. Since a strong immune system is so vital to the long-term prevention of cancer, and since our emotions are so closely linked to the immune system, depression, long-term grief, a sense of hopelessness, or undealt-with emotional conflicts may play a role in the onset of certain cancers. For this and other reasons, the emotional as well as nutritional ways of coping with the onset of cancer do, for the most part, apply to prevention as well. This section, therefore, should be of interest to everyone. I do not have *the* definitive answers; no one does. But I can tell you this: if we believe we can lick it, we are far more likely to do so. Knowing that we can eat and live ourselves out of vulnerability therefore becomes a doubly important factor. Many of my colleagues and I agree that if we could legally avoid using the word *cancer* in diagnosing patients who have it, we could probably save a lot of lives. But the word need not illicit hopelessness and despair—not anymore.

SYMPTOMS

The symptoms of cancer are wide-ranging and may vary from person to person, but there are some common signs to watch for: tiredness, fatigue, unexplained weakness, unexplained mood changes, long-term depression, sudden weight loss, poor appetite, intermittent diarrhea and constipation, blood in stool, recurring unexplained indigestion, back and other aches that persist, abdominal cramps or pain, urinary frequency and/or difficulty, unexplained persisting hoarseness, sores that won't heal, sudden change in a mole on the skin. Self-diagnosis of cancer is, of course, risky, but it is essential that we have enough of an awareness to know when to see our doctor. All too often cancer is not discovered until it is too late to successfully treat.

TREATMENT

Many tumors respond to modern chemotherapeutic chemicals. Some respond to radiation or X-ray treatment. It is, however, becoming increasingly clear that attitude, emotions, and diet play a major role in the treatment (as well as the prevention) of all types of cancer. This means that the treatment of cancer does not end with the doctor's anti-cancer therapy. There is much the patient can do to participate in his or her own recovery in all of these areas.

ANTI-CANCER DIET

Dietary considerations probably relate directly to 35 percent of all cases of cancer, and since the Rejuvenation Diet is an anti-cancer diet, we already have a life-saving foundation. For those of you most concerned about cancer, however, here are further nutritional guidelines.

Since high-fat diets are a direct cause of cancer, anyone serious about preventing or overcoming cancer has another good reason to eliminate these excess fats from the diet. Further evidence, while somewhat inconclusive, exists to suggest that eating large amounts of *polyunsaturated* fats can suppress immunity and may be carcinogenic. You may therefore wish to reduce polyunsaturated fats to levels even lower than Rejuvenation Diet amounts—less than 10 percent of total calories. These can easily be replaced with monounsaturated fats, such as olive oil and borage oil (also known as canola or rapeseed oil), which in moderation do not contribute to causing of cancer but instead appear to strengthen immunity and help in its prevention.

Antioxidant deficiencies have been associated with cancer of the prostate, bladder, colon, liver, and skin. Poor selenium levels have been linked to increased breast, rectal, colon, and prostate cancers. Antioxidants such as beta carotene, vitamin C, and vitamin E have been found to have the ability to capture and neutralize free radicals before they can destroy other cells, and thus may play an important role in the prevention and treatment of cancer. A recent study at Eastern Medical College suggested that beta carotene used together with traditional chemotherapy may have increased success rates in fighting cancer. Vitamin E, another antioxidant, has been seen to stop cancer growths in lab animals.

Since cancer may be due in part to a compromised immune system, we want to make sure we are getting enough vitamin C, selenium, and zinc, as well as beta carotene and vitamin E, all needed for a strong immunity. The thymus gland also plays a role in a healthy immunity, and since the thymus gland uses essential fatty acids (linoleic acid and EPA omega-3) as well as iron, essential amino acids, and vitamins B-6 and B-12, we also want to emphasize these in our anticancer diet.

Other evidence of the role of vitamin E, from the *New England Journal of Medicine,* suggests that low blood levels of this antioxidant are associated with an increased risk of lung cancer, while in a further consideration of beta carotene, researchers found that people who regularly ate leafy green vegetables and yellow vegetables (the best sources of beta carotene) were less likely to develop any and all types of cancers.

Other evidence supporting the need for EPA suggests that omega-3 essential fatty acids, found in most deep-water fish, help to make body chemicals called prostaglandins, some of which rejuvenate T-lymphocyte immunity cells and help produce interferons, both essential in the body's battle against cancer invaders.

Calcium in the diet along with healthy levels of vitamin D have been found to help in the prevention of colon cancer; and fiber in the diet, particularly water-insoluble fiber such as wheat bran and vegetable cellulose, also seems to reduce colon cancer.

Cruciferous vegetables (those in the cabbage family) have begun to emerge as an important ingredient in the dietery fight against cancer, primarily because they are so dense in cancer-fighting nutrients and because they contain indoles (specific chemicals within the plant), which may enhance the body's detoxification abilities. And though the medical jury may still be out on that one, I for one am not going to wait for their verdict. Garlic (whole, not powdered) is another unrecognized but potentially helpful food in the fight against cancer. Since there are no possible harmful effects of either of these yet-to-be-empirically-proven anti-cancer foods, they are certainly worth experimenting with. There is also a somewhat controversial theory that L-lysine, one of the key amino acids, may play an important role in both prevention and treatment of certain cancers. It is now available in supplement form.

But none of these measures will be of much use to us if we are not at a healthy rejuvenation weight. Recent data concluded that men who are 20 percent overweight have a 37 percent greater chance of contracting prostate cancer and a 26 percent greater chance of getting colon cancer; men 40 percent overweight increase the colon cancer risk to 70 percent; women 20 percent overweight increase their risk of uterine cancer by 85 percent, gallbladder cancer by 74 percent, cervical cancer by 50 percent, breast cancer by 16 percent; women 40 percent overweight increase the risk of uterine cancer by 442 percent, gallbladder cancer by 258 percent, cervical cancer by 139 percent, breast cancer by 53 percent, and an overall cancer risk increase of 63 percent. What all this adds up to is that 120,000 people die each year because of what they choose to eat and choose not to eat. And if 35 percent of all cancer is due to diet, with around another 40 percent due to tobacco, consider the preventive power you and I have in our own choices about how to live our lives.

REJUVENATION FOODS TO EMPHASIZE

Leafy green vegetables

All—especially spinach and collards.

Yellow vegetables

All—especially yams, squash, sweet potatoes, pumpkins (with seeds), carrots.

Cruciferous vegetables

Broccoli, cabbage, Brussels sprouts, kale, cauliflower, kohlrabi.

Other vegetables

See the High Fiber List, Rejuvenation Diet.

Fruits

Cantaloupes, fresh strawberries, tomatoes, all citrus, papayas, mangoes, peaches, figs, apricots.

Fish

All fish containing EPA omega-3 (see the Rejuvenation Diet).

Gamma-linoleic acid

Found in: borage (canola or rapeseed) oil, hybrid safflower oil (one teaspoon daily), and evening primrose oil.

Fiber

Forty-plus grams of water insoluble fiber. See the High Fiber List, Rejuvenation Diet.

Other foods

Chestnuts, nonfat yogurt, all legumes, and all high selenium foods—herring, tuna, salmon, mackerel, wheat germ, brewer's yeast.

One or two tablespoons per day of acidophilus liquid to provide a flora of intestinal bacteria, helpful to the body and to the transport of nutrients and immunity throughout the body.

SUPPLEMENTS INCREASED FROM REGULAR REJUVENATION INSURANCE

Though it often goes unnoticed, many people with cancer develop an iron deficiency and should have their doctor perform a serum ferritin test to determine whether an iron supplement is needed. Have him or her check also for a protein deficiency. If needed, increase protein consumption or take amino acid supplements. One thousand micrograms per day of one key amino acid, L-lysine, will also function as an antioxidant by neutralizing free radicals.

For all patients with cancer or a particular concern about its likelihood, I prescribe the following supplementation plan in addition to the basic plan in Chapter 3 (in conjunction with standard medical therapy):

Beta carotene	50,000 IUs daily
B-complex*	150 to 300 mgs (keeping B-6 no higher than 150 mgs) daily
Choline	1000 mcgs daily
Vitamin C	1000 mgs three to six times a day, or to level just before diarrhea
Vitamin D	400 IUs daily
Vitamin E	800 to 1200 IUs daily
Chromium	50 mcgs daily
Magnesium	500 mgs daily
Selenium	100 mcgs daily
Zinc	60 mgs (2 of 30 mgs zinc picolinate) daily
EPA omega-3	300 mgs (in 1000-mg base), one to three capsules daily

*Medical therapy may require the removal of folic acid from B-complex.

THE EXERCISE FACTOR

Exercise stimulates and rejuvenates the entire body and can help in attitude improvement. It is part of all healing programs, cancer included, to the degree that it is safe. Ask your doctor for guidelines.

LIFESTYLE CONSIDERATIONS

Eliminating unnecessary drugs, including cigarettes and coffee, from your life should be a prime consideration, along with the avoidance whenever possible of all potentially carcinogenic substances. This means drinking water without chlorine and other carcinogens, trying to eat produce that has not been permeated with carcinogenic pesticides, not using cosmetics containing formaldehyde, taking direct sunlight only in small amounts, and considering the benefit versus the risk of fluorescent lighting, as well as what to do about the multiple threats we all face from better living with modern chemistry. Upon my suggesting such measures, some of my patients have countered with: "Everything gives you cancer . . . what's the use?" Not true. No one is powerless. Smoking cigarettes is a choice, as is burning one's food or cooking above an open flame. There are cosmetics now available that do not contain harmful substances; osmosis charcoal filters can remove much of the harmful chemicals from water; and there are many ways to improve ventilation where we live and work to decrease the presence of carcinogens in the air we breathe. Spider plants have been found to absorb formaldehyde, for example, and should probably be a part of anyone's collection of house plants. There are a lot of good toxicology books, which I will suggest in the Recommended Reading section, that can help us remove some of the risks from our homes and our lives. And there are still many things in our world that do *not* cause cancer. Listening to Mozart does not cause cancer, nor does swimming in an unpolluted lake, or, for that matter, eating a fresh, organically grown strawberry.

Constipation Plan

IDENTIFICATION AND CAUSES

Constipation is the inability to have more than two bowel movements per week, or having very difficult movements requiring straining. It is a very common problem of people over forty, and like indigestion, it is not a disease but rather a symptom—usually of inadequate fluid intake, inadequate fiber in the diet, food allergies, lack of exercise, and anxiety and/or depression. It may even be due to hormone deficiencies as in hypothyroidism. In some people constipation can even be brought on by ignoring the constant contraction of the colon muscle over a period of time. This usually happens to people who very often find themselves in a public place without restrooms when it is time for a bowel movement, and is known as commuter's constipation.

SYMPTOMS

Infrequent bowel movements, resulting in chronic abdominal fullness and flatus are the predominant symptoms. "Infrequent" can mean many things to many people. This is determined by how often you usually have a bowel movement. While some people normally have one every other day, some normally have two in one day, so there is no certain time formula for what defines constipation for everyone—though preventive cancer therapy would advise at least one bowel movement per day. Occasional constipation can happen to anyone and need not be a major concern. Chronic constipation, however, is a serious matter. It prevents the body from removing carcinogens and other toxins in a safe and timely manner; and besides the bloating and discomfort, over time it can increase the risk of gall bladder disease, colon cancer, and possibly other cancers. If constipation persists for two to three weeks despite changing your diet according to my recommendations, see a doctor, as constipation can in some cases be the symptom of a tumor.

TREATMENT

Medical treatment is necessary to rule out any number of serious accompanying illnesses. Beyond that, however, all too often doctors send their patients home with laxatives. Laxatives treat only the symptom, not the cause, and their side effects range from nutrient malabsorption to skin rashes, gastric irritation, abdominal bloating, and magnesium toxicity. Because they treat symptom and not cause, they can cause addictions. A change in diet, an increase in activity, and perhaps the management of stress and anxiety are essential measures and probably the most effective overall treatment for anyone suffering from constipation.

ANTI-CONSTIPATION DIET

Whether or not you are under medical treatment—unless kidney disease or heart disease treatment dictates otherwise—the treatment of constipation requires lots of water: ten to fourteen glasses a day. Along with that you need lots of fiber (assuming you are not suffering an organ disease, such as colon cancer, ileitis, bowel inflammation disease, or pancreatic disease). Since high fiber is crucial to longevity, consider yourself lucky if a bout with constipation can motivate you in that direction. If you suffer from constipation you probably are not used to a high fiber diet, so I suggest starting with about 20 to 40 grams of fiber per day and working up slowly from there to 60, even 65 grams per day. This should avoid any abdominal gripping, cramping, gassiness, or the general discomfort some people suffer from a sudden leap in their fiber intake level. Most of my patients who need to increase fiber find it easiest if they begin with a high-fiber breakfast, such as any high-fiber, unprocessed cereal garnished with two fresh prunes, two fresh figs, and one tablespoon of wheat bran. I also recommend up to one quart per day of dry popcorn along with an extra emphasis on ten to fourteen glasses a day of filtered water.

There are no specific supplements beyond the regular rejuvenation insurance required to treat or prevent constipation, but I can recommend an anti-constipation drink to have before breakfast:

One cup boiled water, 2 tablespoons blackstrap molasses, and 1/2 lemon squeezed into the water. This mixture changes the bacterial flora in the colon, encouraging the growth of the helpful bacteria we need.

REJUVENATION FOODS TO EMPHASIZE

Whole grains

Oat or wheat bran, any unprocessed (unsalted, unsugared, *non-instant*) whole-grain cereals such as cream of wheat, cream of rice, kasha, puffed wheat, shredded wheat, puffed barley, millet, wheat berries.

Vegetables (best eaten raw, if possible)

Beets, broccoli, Brussels sprouts, carrots, cauliflower, corn, greens (especially collard and beet greens), green peas, pumpkins, baked potatoes, sweet potatoes, baked yams (with skins).

Legumes

Lima beans, chick peas (garbanzo beans), kidney beans, pinto beans, lentils, soybeans.

Fruits

Apples, pears, bananas.

Nuts and seeds

Peanuts, chestnuts, unsalted roasted soy beans, sunflower seeds, psyllium seeds, almonds, millet, sesame.

THE EXERCISE FACTOR

Exercise is a must. A forty-minute walk per day can sometimes be a complete cure for constipation—though keep up your high-fiber diet for a number of other health reasons. A change in diet, however, without adding some sort of rigorous activity may not achieve the desired result.

LIFESTYLE CONSIDERATIONS

If the cause is stress-related, see the Stress Plan. If you suffer from commuter's constipation, you may have to rearrange your life slightly to accommodate your elimination system. It is crucial to your health.

Cystitis Plan

IDENTIFICATION AND CAUSES

For many people cystitis, also known as urinary tract infection (UTI), is, quite simply, a bacterial infection of the bladder resulting in a number of uncomfortable symptoms. Urinary tract infections are usually caused by chemical irritants, bacterial invasion, or allergic reactions, but they can also be instigated by inadequate fluid consumption and from wearing tight-fitting nylon underwear or outer garments. Baths are another common cause, since we are sitting relaxed in dirty water which can easily float up the urinary tract. Another is sexual intercourse with a partner who is unclean. Sexual transmission and prostate enlargement are the two major causes for men, but cystitis is generally a women's health concern.

Women are at far greater risk than men since their urinary tracts are much shorter, and since rectal bacteria can easily enter the urethra and cause infection. I have even seen a woman who got recurrent cystitis from a contraceptive diaphram that was too tight. Women over forty seem to be at the greatest risk of contracting a urinary tract infection. Their bodies produce less estrogen, which causes shrinkage of urinary tract tissues and results in inadequate urinary drainage and urine stagnation in the bladder. Urinary tract infections, in men and women, can also occur when an infected kidney sends bacteria down to the bladder.

SYMPTOMS

Burning during urination, a foul odor in the urine, and frequency and urgency of urination are the most universal symptoms of this painful and treatable disorder. A fever may accompany any or all of these symptoms, which warrant investigation by a urologist.

TREATMENT

A visit to the urologist is necessary, first to rule out another disease such as diabetes, kidney problems, or yeast infection, and then to determine the cause. If it is an allergy, treatment will likely consist of avoiding the allergen and taking antibiotics. For most women over forty, the problem will often clear up after the urethra has been stretched, allowing for easier and freer urinary flow. There are also certain foods and supplements we can take to expedite recovery while under the care of a competent urologist.

ANTI-CYSTITIS DIET

The cranberry juice treatment is no longer just folklore. Recent scientific evidence found that the metabolites, which are breakdown products of digested cranberry juice, acidify urine and actually prevent bacteria from adhering to the wall of the bladder. To put it plainly, the bacteria do not like cranberry juice. Three to four 8-ounce glasses of cranberry juice (without added sugar) is a good daily dosage. The other crucial ingredient for recovery—or prevention—of this painful syndrome is lots of water: ten to fourteen 8-ounce glasses per day. Other juices, fruit and vegetable (no added sugar or salt*) as well as unsalted* soups will also help.

There are also two nutrients that I have found useful in treating cystitis. Beta carotene is good for maintaining the integrity of the mucus tissues. Vitamin C, I have discovered, can also help to acidify urine and to protect against bacteria.

REJUVENATION FOODS TO EMPHASIZE

Vegetables

Leafy greens, dark greens, yellow and orange, shiitake mushrooms.

---

*Since most low-sodium vegetable juices and soups taste quite horrid to most people, you may want to invest in a juicer and enjoy your juices and soups fresh and homemade.

Fruits

All citrus fruits.

Whole grains

Brown rice, wheat germ.

Legumes

Soybeans.

SUPPLEMENTS INCREASED FROM REGULAR REJUVENATION INSURANCE

Beta carotene	10,000 IUs daily
Vitamin C	1000 mgs, three times a day

THE EXERCISE FACTOR

While exercise is crucial to everyone's good health, there is no specific indication that it has any direct effect on prevention or treatment of urinary infections other than fortifying of the immune system.

LIFESTYLE CONSIDERATIONS

No baths. Lolling in a tub encourages bacteria to enter the urinary opening. Take showers, at least until the infection goes away, and if recurring infections persist, consider a permanent change to showers. If currently using nylon underwear, switch to cotton and avoid polyester outer garments as well. Women should always wipe from front to back, never the other way. Reduce alcohol, and if you use diuretics to keep your weight down, stop immediately.

Depression Plan

IDENTIFICATION AND CAUSES

Depression is perhaps the most common—and certainly the most underdiagnosed—illness encountered by today's physician. Difficult to define in medical terms, though any physician knows it when he sees it, depression can be described as "withdrawal from life" or "mental and physical apathy." As many as one in five patients who enters a doctor's office suffers from depression. Depressions can be caused by a vast assortment of psychological and physical conditions; there are probably as many causes for depression as there are possible physical symptoms. In fact, it is often difficult to identify whether a depression is the cause or result of any number of physical illnesses. In this plan I limit myself to the physical aspects of depression; psychological causes, such as anxiety or mourning, are too complex for this book and are not my field of expertise.

Common physical causes of depression range from hormonal imbalances, such as the menstrual cycle, hypothyroidism, PMS, and menopause to diabetes and low blood sugar. Very often, I have found, depression is a reaction to food, and recent medical literature on allergies has confirmed my suspicions. Excess caffeine and sugar consumption can bring on severe depression, as can vitamin deficiencies, especially of the B vitamins. Many food colorings, additives, and other chemicals have been found to bring on depression in certain people. Chlorine, lead, cadmium, and other toxic metals—present in the water from the average American tap—can produce all sorts of mood swings, including depression.

SYMPTOMS

Depression can affect any and every part of the human body. It can bring on—and be masked by—chronic headaches, recurring abdominal pains, recurring backache, and chronic diffuse pains (pains throughout the body, often shooting pains, difficult to identify). The symptoms of depression are perhaps the most wide-ranging of any illness. Virtually any syndrome in this book can be, at least to some degree, the result of a depression.

TREATMENT

The most important information you can give your doctor is an awareness of your depression and of its possible nature. If emotional causes seem unlikely, then determining the physical cause of the depression will probably determine the treatment. There is, however, no standard practice established in medicine for treating depression other than prescriptive drugs, some of which are successful but carry side effects.

If the cause of the depression is physical, a check of the endocrine system is needed to rule out a thyroid imbalance. An allergy workup also is in order, considering foods, medications, chemicals in air and water, clothes, and other contactants. I once had a patient who mysteriously got depressed every Sunday. At first she assumed it was some childhood remembrance of dreading the return to school every Monday morning, but as the depression grew worse and worse, she was checked for every food allergy plus a hundred other environmental factors. She was considering psychotherapy by the time she came to me. I asked her what she did differently on Sundays than on other days. "I read the paper in bed," she informed me. "I guess the news depresses me." But it wasn't the news. It turned out that she was allergic to the colored ink on the Sunday comics. It got on her hands, into her bloodstream, and it made her depressed. Realizing this, she had her husband pick up the Sunday paper and tried putting it in the oven for fifteen minutes at a low setting to bake off the colored ink. It worked. Now, when she reads the comics, she laughs.

A depression can also be the result of a mild anemia, and a blood-serum ferritin test may save you years of therapy.

Sometimes the cause of a depression can be emotional as well as physical, so nothing must be ruled out until both illness and symptom have been alleviated. In the meantime, however, there are some nutritional anti-depression measures effective for depressions of all kinds.

ANTI-DEPRESSION DIET

Calcium and magnesium are natural anti-depressants for some people. Additionally, there are specific foods that, for somewhat mysterious reasons, often help people overcome the symptoms of a depression while they are treating the root cause.

REJUVENATION FOODS TO EMPHASIZE

Vegetables

All green vegetables, all root vegetables.

Fruits

Bananas, mangoes.

All nonfat dairy products.

All whole grains.

Fish

Sardines, salmon, shellfish.

Other protein sources

White meat turkey, soybean products, cashews and almonds.

SUPPLEMENTS INCREASED FROM REGULAR REJUVENATION INSURANCE

L-tryptophan	500 mg four times daily, in association with:
Vitamin B-6	25 mg (with each L-tryptophan dosage)
Niacin*	50 mg (with each L-tryptophan dosage)
B-complex	200 mg daily
Vitamin C**	1000 mg four or five times daily
Calcium	1500 mg total daily
Magnesium	1000 mg total daily
Zinc	30 mg total daily

DL-phenylalanine, an amino acid, may also help relieve depression, but must be taken under a doctor's supervision; it has been observed to have a reverse effect in some people.

---

*If niacin causes flushes, replace with niacinamide, 50 to 100 mg per dosage.
**If 4000 to 5000 mg of vitamin C causes diarrhea, decrease dosage to comfortable amount.

THE EXERCISE FACTOR

There are very few depressed joggers—or regular brisk walkers. I have also prescribed t'ai chi to depressed patients, with considerable results. See Chapter 5.

LIFESTYLE CONSIDERATIONS

Psychotherapy may be in order, or perhaps just a bit of self-honesty. Mozart or Schubert therapy works for some people, as does listening to cassette tapes of Gregorian chants.

Diabetes Plan

IDENTIFICATION AND CAUSES

Diabetes, an inability of the body to process its blood sugar, is usually caused by a pancreatic inability to produce sufficient insulin. Since fat metabolism can only occur properly if the liver can burn carbohydrate fuel adequately, and since insulin is needed for that function, diabetes also means an inability to metabolize fat. Diabetes can cause blood sugar to rise to unsafe levels, risking coma and death. Causes of diabetes may include genetic virus; the excess demands of obesity on the body; or cells in the body that fail to accept, recognize, or utilize insulin.

There are two common types of diabetes, known simply as Type I and Type II diabetes; neither has been linked definitively to a cause.

Type I (also known as insulin-dependent diabetes because the patient is unable to produce insulin in the body) tends to strike younger people—it is sometimes called juvenile diabetes, though we are discovering that it is quite possible for those over forty to develop this disorder. One current theory is that it is caused by a viral infection; other theories maintain that Type I diabetes is a genetic predisposition aggravated by a viral infection.

Type II, also called non–insulin dependent or adult-onset diabetes, is the type most likely to occur in those over forty. While it has not yet been established that excess refined sugars and refined carbohydrates, excess fats, and excess calories in general cause diabetes, there is no doubt that these destructive foods and eating habits make the condition much worse once it exists. In fact, obesity can make the control of diabetes nearly impossible, blocking the body's cells from absorbing or using badly needed insulin. There are also emotional factors connected with this condition. Duress and stress commonly elevate blood sugars and blood lipids, which further worsen diabetes.

SYMPTOMS

Commonly associated with both kinds of diabetes are fatigue, itchy skin, frequent urination, nighttime urination, weight loss from excess water loss and a metabolism gone haywire, extreme appetite swings, muscle weakening, tingling neuropathies, tingling neuritis of hands and legs, hair loss, various skin lesions, dermatitis, high blood pressure, heart irregularities, kidney and bladder infections, poor healing of wounds, headaches, and vision problems. Since many of these symptoms can be caused by disorders other than diabetes, and since diabetes greatly increases the risk of heart attacks, strokes, infections, and suppressed immunity, it is important that you be examined by your doctor to determine if you have diabetes.

TREATMENT

Treating diabetes is very much a medical matter, requiring strict adherence to your physician's recommendations. I also urge you, if you are diagnosed as diabetic, to have your cholesterol—HDL, LDL, and VLDL—checked and, if they are high, please see the High Cholesterol Plan to get that under control, as diabetics are at extremely high risk for arteriosclerosis and heart attacks.

There are also some dietary and exercise measures you can take that will expedite—and are essential to—the treatment of diabetes.

ANTI-DIABETES DIET

Almost all diabetics need to lose weight (see the Obesity and Addiction Plans for specifics). In addition—and helpful to the weight-losing cause—diabetics must completely eliminate alcohol, refined sugars and carbohydrates, and saturated fats (this means no fried or processed foods) while reducing other fats to levels even lower than recommended in the Rejuvenation Diet: 10 to 15 percent (not 20 percent) of total calories consumed (about one tablespoon daily of total oil). Protein should account for about 12 percent of all calories (or no more than 40 grams per day, which equals 3.5 ounces of halibut, one baked sweet potato, and 6 ounces of snow peas), and the rest should be complex carbohydrates. Whenever possible, eat your vegetables and fruits raw rather than cooked—this seems to be less burdensome to the pancreas—and limit certain complex carbohydrates that are dense in complex sugars (listed below).

Emphasize fiber in your diet, consuming 25 grams of fiber for every 1000 calories. This means about 40 to 50 grams daily, which means unprocessed whole grain cereal for breakfast and lots of high fiber vegetables throughout the day. Fiber not only helps lower insulin need but the bulk provided by fiber also helps lower caloric intake and relieves the extreme hunger experienced by some diabetics.

You may want to consider these recent nutritional findings: some essential oils retard arteriosclerosis and thus may be helpful to the diabetic; a chromium supplement may help stabilize blood sugar; and zinc, an essential part of the insulin molecule, also seems to help diabetics heal better when taken in supplemental form along with vitamin C.

REJUVENATION FOODS TO LIMIT

fruit	2 daily
carrots	1 large daily
sweet potato or yam	1 medium daily
protein	12% of total calories (or no more than 40 grams daily
fats	15% of total calories daily

REJUVENATION FOODS TO EMPHASIZE

All whole grains.

All nonfat dairy.

All cruciferous vegetables

Broccoli, Brussels sprouts, cabbage, cauliflower, kohlrabi, kale.

All legumes.

All EPA-containing fish. (See the Rejuvenation Diet)

Oils

Olive oil, borage (canola) oil (1 to 2 teaspoons daily).

SUPPLEMENTS INCREASED FROM REGULAR REJUVENATION INSURANCE

Vitamin C*	6000 mgs daily
GTF Chromium**	100 mcgs daily
Zinc picolinate**	30 mgs twice daily

THE EXERCISE FACTOR

Daily exercise relieves diabetes and is a necessary part of treatment. Recent studies have indicated that, even without a restricted diet, diabetics can elevate insulin levels through a regular exercise program. Exercise for the diabetic is an aerobic, seven-day-a-week commitment of about an hour per day. Exercise of this kind appears to balance the metabolism of all fuels, improve the absorption of amino acids from protein, and improve metabolism of fatty acids and glucose—though no one has yet determined why.

*Vitamin C can make some blood sugar treatments difficult and should be considered with your physician
**Chromium and zinc should always be taken together

Exercise drastically changes insulin requirements in anyone with diabetes, so it must always be done under the supervision of a doctor.

LIFESTYLE CONSIDERATIONS

Since stress can aggravate diabetes, stress management and a change in attitude are essential. See the Stress Plan.

Diverticulosis Plan

IDENTIFICATION AND CAUSES

Diverticulosis refers to a condition in which small pouches, called diverticula, form on the inner surface of the colon. Food gets trapped in these pouches and ferments, causing the diverticula to become irritated, inflamed, and sometimes abscessed. Many experts refer to diverticulosis as "the disease of modern American civilization," as it seems to be directly related to a diet of low-fiber refined foods. (Studies of African societies known to eat high-crude–fiber diets showed almost no cases of diverticulosis.) The disease takes many years to manifest, so most cases of diverticulosis occur in people in their forties and fifties.

SYMPTOMS

This syndrome may cause alternating diarrhea and constipation, agonizing bouts of gas, and/or pain on the left side of the abdomen. But often diverticulosis goes unnoticed and is diagnosed by a physician for some unrelated reason during an examination of the large intestines. If not diagnosed in time, however, a host of very noticeable symptoms may occur: inflammation will cause extreme abdominal pain and may be accompanied by vomiting, fever, and/or rectal bleeding. If any or all of these symptoms beset you, call your doctor immediately. If not treated, this condition can cause a rupture of the colon.

TREATMENT

Medical treatment by a doctor, usually requiring antibiotics and a change in diet, is the only way to alleviate this condition. My own recommendations should not differ from those of your own physician.

ANTI-DIVERTICULOSIS DIET

Diverticulosis is a disorder directly related to diet. Both prevention and treatment are dependent on changes in the diet. We need to cut way down on all refined sugars and refined carbohydrates, and eliminate saturated fats. There are also some "real" foods we must avoid as long as we have the condition. Berries, figs, nuts, all seeds, and popcorn have tiny indigestible pieces that can get trapped inside the diverticula and further obstruct these pouches. We need to start eating 40 to 50 grams per day of fiber, mostly water insoluble, and to include acidophilus as part of our daily consumption to reduce putrefying types of bacteria.

REJUVENATION FOODS TO EMPHASIZE

Whole grains (can be eaten as unprocessed cereal and unprocessed bread)

Wheat, oat, rye, rice (about 28 grams of fiber per ounce).

Vegetables

Spinach, cabbage, cauliflower, potatoes, sweet potatoes (with skin), yams (with skin).

Legumes

All beans (about 10 grams of fiber per cup).

SUPPLEMENTS INCREASED FROM REGULAR REJUVENATION INSURANCE

Acidophilus liquid	1 to 3 tbsp daily

THE EXERCISE FACTOR

Exercise is crucial for normal colon function. Abdominal muscle motion massages the colon, encouraging more rapid emptying of the colon, and reducing putrefaction. There are no special exercises you must do; walking forty minutes to an hour daily is most effective.

LIFESTYLE CONSIDERATIONS

See Chapter 6.

Emphysema Plan

IDENTIFICATION AND CAUSES

This lung disorder, medically known as chronic obstructive pulmonary disease (or COPD), is the most common lung problem in men and women over forty. It is characterized by enlargement of the air spaces in the lungs, usually at the ends of the lungs, accompanied by the destruction of these walls and the loss of lung elasticity. The collapse of the organ tissue obliterates the airways, causing great difficulty in the expiration of air from the lungs. The cause is chronic infection of the lungs brought on by any number of provocative agents, especially cigarette smoke (active or passive) and various air pollutants. It is a progressive illness, usually beginning early in a person's life, though symptoms are usually not present until the age of forty to fifty.

SYMPTOMS

The earliest signs of emphysema may be a mild (almost unrecognized) cough, weight loss, weakness, or loss of libido. As the disease progresses, the most common complaint is shortness of breath on exertion. Wheezing and recurring infections may also result. If you suspect that you might be in the early to middle stages of this illness, if you smoke, or if you live in a polluted city, you may want to test your exhaling capacity.

This can be done quite easily: take a deep breath and exhale as fast as possible, clocking how long it takes to remove all the air from the lungs. If it takes much more than about four seconds, see your doctor.

TREATMENT

There is no known cure for emphysema—that is, there is no way yet devised for reversing the disease—but modern medicine has developed many ways to treat the symptoms and stop further progression. A physician is needed to perform X rays and possibly pulmonary function testing to determine whether in fact you have emphysema, and if you test positive, to give you the best available treatment. There are, however, one dietary and a few lifestyle considerations I can recommend for anyone with this illness.

ANTI-EMPHYSEMA DIET

Since the Rejuvenation Diet is an immunity-fortifying diet, adherence to it may decrease the likelihood of recurring lung infections and will keep the emphysema from weakening you to point of vulnerability to other diseases. In addition, time and again beta carotene and vitamin E have proven to be lung protective and may be useful both to the person fighting the progression of emphysema and to the person who lives in Los Angeles or Mexico City, or who lives with a smoker.

REJUVENATION FOODS TO EMPHASIZE

Beta carotene foods

All fish, green and yellow vegetables (especially broccoli, kale, and carrots), green and yellow fruits (especially apricots and avocados), nonfat dairy.

Vitamin E foods

Dark green vegetables, wheat germ, brown rice, soybeans.

SUPPLEMENTS INCREASED FROM REGULAR REJUVENATION INSURANCE

Beta carotene	25,000 IUs daily
Vitamin E	600 to 800 IUs daily

THE EXERCISE FACTOR

Aerobic exercise helps to restimulate healing in the lung and is therefore of tremendous importance. Consult your physician to determine how much you should do per day, and if you choose walking or jogging, make an extra effort to do it where you will not be breathing heavily polluted air.

LIFESTYLE CONSIDERATIONS

Since lifestyle choices are probably the major contributing factor in the onset of emphysema, these choices may very well dictate the management of this illness. Smoking and being around people who smoke are no longer affordable luxuries. Most of us who live in major metropolitan centers of air pollution cannot pick up and leave at will, but there are other measures we can take to ensure that what we breathe is as clean as possible. Breathing through the nose is a good place to start; the nose is the best natural air filtration system we have. Proper ventilation and clean air-conditioning ducts are certainly within our control. And the measures we take may save a loved one from developing the same problem later in life.

Epstein-Barr Virus Plan

IDENTIFICATION AND TREATMENT

This virus, cousin of the herpes virus, has only very recently leaped out of obscurity to become a considerable health concern to an increasing number of people. Epstein-Barr virus infection, as the term is used today, refers to a mysterious type of chronic mononucleosis. The latest findings by The National Cancer Institute suggest it may be brought on by a newly discovered human B-lymphotrophic herpes virus (HBLV). God only knows where HBLV came from. It is a significant illness; and because it is such a recent phenomenon, many cases have gone undiagnosed, sometimes leaving the victim (and the victim's friends and family) believing he or she is going insane or is at least becoming a hypochondriac. I have, in fact, been surprised to see several patients relieved to be told they had Epstein-Barr, just to know there was something responsible for their symptoms. It is not an age-related illness, but one of which we must nonetheless beware. A past bout with mononucleosis does not increase the risk of contracting Epstein-Barr, but a weak immunity does.

SYMPTOMS

Thus far in its brief existence the Epstein-Barr virus has been known to cause profound fatigue, weakness, recurring sore throats, severe depression, extreme mood swings, recurring fever and chills, appetite swings, muscle aches and pains, and, in some cases, enlarged and tender lymph nodes.

TREATMENT

There is as yet no certain treatment for this virus, though there is much research going on, especially with a herpes treatment drug known as Acyclovir. You will want to make sure your physician is up on all the latest findings so that he can offer you the best possible treatment.

ANTI–EPSTEIN-BARR VIRUS DIET

Since this viral illness may be an autoimmune disease and is, at the very least, an illness that afflicts people with a lowered immunity, the Rejuvenation Diet, a diet for strengthening immunity, is your best therapy. The most serious dietary consideration if you are suffering from Epstein-Barr is not to allow any diminished appetite to prevent good nutrition, which will slow down recovery. Supplements should include those recommended in Chapter 3, along with suggested increases from the Herpes Plan.

THE EXERCISE FACTOR

In moderation, exercise can be an important part of recovery, as it helps raise immunity against this and other viruses. But be careful to stay within the limitations imposed by your body signals. Do not exercise when severely ill.

LIFESTYLE CONSIDERATIONS

As with all immune diseases, the mind has a profound influence. Undealt-with anger and other negative emotions can land you in a hospital bed. See Chapter 6 and the Herpes Plan.

Fibrocystic Breast Disease Plan

IDENTIFICATION AND CAUSES

There are two significant types of breast disease which concern most women: benign fibrocystic breast disease (noncancerous and treatable) and breast cancer. Both can be characterized by a variety of different types of growths, 80 percent to 90 percent of which are fortunately not cancerous. Sometimes benign breast disease can be part of the symptoms of premenstrual syndrome and will come and go with a woman's cycle. Sometimes the lumps and other symptoms will go away without treatment, but since there is always the possibility of an underlying breast cancer, nothing out of the ordinary should go unreported to a physician.

Fibrocystic disease, also known as mammary dysplasia and chronic cystic mastitis, which is most likely to affect women of forty-five and under, can nevertheless strike any woman at any time; and breast cancer, which is a concern of women at any age, may occur as the result of many factors, including heredity. But more and more research and data points to the diet as a significant factor. Excess fat consumption is now clearly linked to increased risk of breast disease, and another recent study discovered a 40 percent greater incidence of breast disease in women who drink four or more alcoholic drinks per day. Everything a woman ingests passes through her breast fluids within a few minutes. Nearly ten years ago a study was published showing a decrease in benign breast disease in women who eliminated from their diets the chemicals caffeine and methylxanthine (and its relatives), commonly found in chocolate, coffee, cola drinks, and tea. Since then, other studies have linked coffee consumption to breast disease. Smoking cigarettes has also been implicated recently.

SYMPTOMS

Fibrocystic breast disease is often detected by the patient in a self-examination. The symptoms are commonly swelling and pain in the breasts, sometimes accompanied by solid lumpy patches, cysts (lumps filled with fluid), or other kinds of growths. These symptoms can sometimes indicate the possibility of breast cancer, but recent studies have found that all too often there are no early signs of breast cancer. It is therefore crucial for all women near or over forty to have a mammogram every year; I urge women over fifty to have one every six months.

TREATMENT

Fibrocystic breast disease is often treated with hormones or diuretics. These I consider to be somewhat extreme measures or last resort tactics. If your physician suggests hormone therapy or diuretics, ask if there are alternatives, and have your thyroid checked. Hypothyroidism can often cause the onset of lumpy painful breasts.

Breast cancer requires multiple therapies depending upon size and spread. Lumpectomy, radiation, and chemotherapy may be necessary. See the Cancer Plan for diet.

ANTI-FIBROCYSTIC BREAST DISEASE DIET

With evidence mounting about the connection between dietary fat and breast disease, your Rejuvenation Diet already tries to eliminate saturated and most polyunsaturated fats. If you feel that you are at high risk for breast disease—for example, if your mother or a sister has already had a bout with breast disease—you may want to further diminish fat. Cutting down drastically on salt will decrease water retention and may alleviate breast swelling, and it will certainly eliminate any need for diuretics. You will also want to abstain completely from alcohol, chocolate, coffee, cola, and tea. Beyond that there are no foods in particular you will need to emphasize; just follow a healthy Rejuvenation Diet.

SUPPLEMENTS INCREASED FROM REGULAR REJUVENATION INSURANCE

I have discovered that breast lumpiness diminishes in many women who consume extra vitamin E. Since this vitamin in large doses can cause high blood pressure, I am careful to start dosages at 100 to 400 IUs, increasing to 600 IUs; if you decide to try this, do so with the supervision of your doctor. As breast cysts and discomfort recede, I reduce dosage back down to 200 to 400 IUs.

I have also been impressed by the evidence on beta carotene in the prevention or control of noncancerous breast tumors. I like to prescribe 25,000 IUs per day.

Vitamin B-1 and thiamin deficiencies can also cause breast swelling and lumpiness, and I recommend 30 milligrams of B-1 and 100 milligrams of thiamin per day to any woman suffering from these symptoms.

For those of you who feel you are at particular risk of breast cancer, or just want an extra precaution against it, selenium may help. A recent University of San Diego study found that in those parts of the world where breast cancer was the lowest, selenium content in the soil was the highest. Selenium may also prove helpful in the prevention and treatment of noncancerous tumors; and though its use remains somewhat controversial, the weight of evidence begins to support its need in the diet of any woman concerned about breast disease. I recommend 50 to 100 micrograms of organic selenium daily, which will work best if taken with at least 100 IUs of vitamin E.

THE EXERCISE FACTOR

There are no specific exercises that help to prevent and treat breast disease. If you do have fibrocystic disease or breast cancer, and if upper body movement is somewhat painful, you will, of course, want to restrict activity; but remember that walking forty minutes to an hour a day, which need not involve the upper body, is all you need.

LIFESTYLE CONSIDERATIONS

See Chapter 6.

Chronic Headache Plan

IDENTIFICATION AND CAUSES

A chronic headache can strike anyone at any age, not the least of who may be those of us over forty. There are basically three types of headaches, any of which may be experienced either chronically or periodically by anyone: type one, scalp contraction, usually referred to as tension headache, is caused by contracting of the scalp and/or neck; type two, vascular headache, is caused by dilation and spasming of blood vessels within the scalp and/or brain (migraine and other cluster headaches are examples); type three, sinus headache, is caused by an infection of the sinus lining or an obstruction of the sinus outlet.

Like many other common conditions, headaches are not a disease but rather a symptom of any number of possible illnesses: General illness, allergies of all kinds (to substances of all kinds), stress, anemia, excess alcohol, caffeine (and caffeine withdrawals), tobacco, and low or high blood sugar are all common causes of headaches. So are nutrient deficiencies; excess vitamin A (which is why vitamin A should always be taken as its precursor, beta carotene); prescription and over-the-counter medications; preservatives such as sulfates, nitrites, and monosodium glutamate (MSG); artificial sweetners such as aspartame; polluting chemicals; fermented cheeses; and certain amino acids such as tyrosine, found in fermented cheese and wine.

SYMPTOMS

One thing all headaches have in common is pain. Where they differ is in the kind of pain and, sometimes, in the intensity of the pain.

Scalp contraction headaches cause general tight pressure or sharp contracting pain. Of the vascular headaches, migraines can be associated with nausea, vomiting, depression, and scotoma—seeing flashing lights—which can lead to photophobia and throbbing or piercing pain. Cluster headaches, usually occurring in men, cause excruciating pain, usually on one side of the head. Sinus headaches cause heavy pressurized pain.

TREATMENT

Identifying both the type and cause of headache is crucial. In many cases this alone will lead to immediate and effective treatment. It will likely require a physician and/or allergist. If treatment does not bring immediate relief, there are many pain-reducing medications available, but they all have side effects. Since they do not treat the cause, they do not lessen the condition; some may, in the long run, worsen the condition or cause other, different headaches. Before you take any drugs, whether prescription or OTC, make sure to ask your doctor if there are alternatives. The Rejuvenation Diet and supplementation insurance along with daily exercise and stress management will help and may in some cases be all the treatment needed. If not, the temporary use of certain painkillers may be valuable if their effect on such debilitating pain outweighs their negative side effects. Long-term use of painkillers, however, knocks out our own brain opiates (the endorphins), making headaches more painful and more difficult to overcome.

ANTI-HEADACHE DIET

If you are a chronic headache victim, I urge you to stop consuming caffeine; the temporary withdrawal headaches will be worth enduring to eradicate the chronic caffeine headaches. Cutting out caffeine involves watching out for all foods and medications containing this drug. Also avoid alcohol, fermented cheeses, chocolate, and nitrites and sulfates found in cured meats and bacon, at least until they can be ruled out as causes. Also avoid artificial food colors, especially yellow dye #5 and sodium benzoate. If you have already decided to extend your life-span by following the Rejuvenation Diet, these measures should not at all be drastic. There are also some rejuvenation foods and some supplements you may wish to emphasize. They are foods high in essential fatty acids which are now known to produce anti-inflammatory prostaglandins.

REJUVENATION FOODS TO EMPHASIZE

Fish

All deep-water EPA omega-3–containing fish (fresh, unprocessed). See the Rejuvenation Diet.

Oils

Olive oil, borage (canola or rapeseed) oil, hybrid safflower oil.*

SUPPLEMENTS INCREASED FROM REGULAR REJUVENATION INSURANCE**

Vitamin C	4000 to 6000 mgs daily, divided up throughout the day
Vitamin E	800 IUs daily
EPA omega-3	300 mgs (in 1000-mg base), three capsules per day
DL-phenylalanine†	500 mgs, three times per day (on an empty stomach) for 7 days; then 500 mgs once per day for 3 weeks; after that, 500 mgs per day for one week of each month
L-tryptophan‡	2000 mgs at bedtime for one week; thereafter, 1000 mgs at bedtime

*These oils should be consumed in small amounts (1 to 3 teaspoons per day) and should never be heated.

**If headache is stress-related, see the Stress Plan for additional supplemental increase.

†Use DL-phenylalanine with your doctor's approval, and never use it if you have high blood pressure.

‡Do not use L-tryptophan if you have liver disease; have your doctor measure your blood liver function.

THE EXERCISE FACTOR

Since exercise relieves stress, it can be a major aid in stopping certain headaches. If the headache is not stress-related, exercise of increased intensity (your doctor permitting) can release endorphins in the body, which are natural painkillers. In general, try not to allow a chronic headache to prevent at least a daily walk. Sometimes the fresh air alone can be extremely valuable.

LIFESTYLE CONSIDERATIONS

Eliminating potential trigger causes of headaches must become a priority, regardless of any inconvenience this causes. Stress management is also essential. Even if the headache is not stress-induced, a headache can cause stress which can worsen the condition. (See the Stress Plan.) Try hatha yoga and biofeedback. Massage and cold packs on the forehead may stop early headaches, especially migraines. A headache may just be nature's way of telling you to take better care of your mind, body, and spirit. Listen.

Heart Disease Plan

IDENTIFICATION AND CAUSES

It is no secret that heart disease is the number one killer of Americans, especially those over forty. Nearly 20 percent of all Americans suffer from heart disease. The vast majority of them do not have to, and can reverse their condition starting immediately. Heart disease is not an illness but an entire category, a class unto itself, covering a large variety of illnesses that affect the heart. Some are congenital and some hereditary. But most heart diseases are caused by enlargement of the heart, vessel obstruction in the heart, failure of the heart muscle or pump action efficiency, calcification and distortion of heart valves, and lack of oxygenation of the heart tissue. Most of these can be traced to dietary abuse, lack of aerobic exercise, stress, and other personality factors.

SYMPTOMS

The most common *nonspecific* symptoms of heart disease are shortness of breath, tiredness and fatigue, chest pain, edema (swelling of the legs and feet due to water retention), and irregular heartbeats often recognized as palpitations. These irregular beats or palpitations can often be significant and life-threatening if the heart slows down to a virtual standstill. They must receive immediate medical attention, as must the other symptoms. Often people view swelling of the ankles as symptomatic of arthritis. This may be, but the risk that it is a heart problem requires that you check with your physician. Sometimes these symptoms can turn out to be a response to thyroid irregularities, anemia, excess salt in the body, lung disorders, or drug toxicities of aspirin, certain asthma medicines, or even certain heart medicines themselves. Viral infections can also mimic the symptoms of heart disease, as can depression and general anxiety, including the fear associated with being told that you might have a heart problem. But you need a doctor to confirm or to rule out these possibilities.

TREATMENT

No cardiac therapy should ever be conducted without the close supervision of a physician and/or cardiac specialist. First you can expect your doctor to explore the state of your coronary arteries by doing an EKG, a treadmill test, radio isotope studies (commonly known as thallium scan tests), echocardiograms, and dye studies (known as coronary angiograms). These tests will check the blood flow, heart muscle status, and the heart's capacity to meet the demands of your body.

The medicines most commonly used by doctors in the treatment of heart illnesses are diuretics, which remove salt and water from the body, decreasing blood pressure and the volume of blood the heart has to push. For chest pain, doctors often still prescribe nitroglycerin, taken under the tongue, as well as the more modern (though not necessarily always better) calcium–channel-blockers and beta-blocker medicines (which open heart blood vessels), and operations or bypasses.

To increase the efficiency of heart muscle contraction or to control rhythm, digitalis medications are frequently used. These medications all have side effects (see Chapter 4), but are often so necessary and even life-saving that they are worth the temporary side effects they produce.

There is a new and very exciting discovery in the field of treating heart disease, found in a recent study to produce a 50 percent higher survival rate in congestive heart failure patients. It is a chemical found in spinach, peanuts, sardines, and beef, called co-enzyme-Q. It is an essential nutrient, supplying a biochemical spark that creates cellular energy in the body. Recent studies have found that without co-enzyme-Q, various bodily mechanisms, not the least of which may be the heart muscle, can begin to fail. Another study found that co-enzyme-Q controls the flow of oxygen within individual cells in our bodies. Japan and the Soviet Union are already successfully using it to treat heart disease, and it may only be a matter of time before the FDA catches up, approving it for medical use in the United States. In the meantime it is available as a supplement in many vitamin stores.

While I recommend its use, I do so with the qualification that study is not yet completed and, most important, that it is not a panacea. It is not *the* answer to the heart disease, just as a pacemaker, which can save the life of someone with a dangerously irregular heart rhythm, is not the totality of the solution.

The only long-term cure—and the only reliable prevention your physician will probably point out to you—is in the choices you make in the foods you consume and the way you choose to live your life. For many people this reality offers the relief and assurance that they are not suddenly helpless but still very much in command.

ANTI-HEART ATTACK DIET

In the Rejuvenation Diet I recommend the elimination of caffeine, excess saturated fats, excess refined sugars and refined carbohydrates, excess sodium, excess alcohol, and excess calories. If you have heart disease this is no longer a recommendation: it is an ultimatum. If you do not start feeding yourself in a healthy manner you will be very sick and may die soon. The rejuvenation foods to emphasize are the same as in the High Cholesterol and Hypertension Plans, plus those foods found to be highest in co-enzyme-Q. There are also some supplements you may wish to use under the supervision of your physician, including the newest breakthrough, co-enzyme-Q.

REJUVENATION FOODS TO EMPHASIZE

Co-enzyme-Q foods

Sardines,* spinach, peanuts.

SUPPLEMENTS INCREASED FROM REGULAR REJUVENATION INSURANCE

L-carnitine**	500 mgs, two capsules daily
Niacin	25 mgs, four times a day, working up to 100 mgs four times a day
EPA omega-3†	300 mgs (in 1000-mg base), one capsule twice a day, working up to three times a day
Co-enzyme-Q	20 mgs, twice a day

THE EXERCISE FACTOR

There is no better heart therapy than regular aerobic exercise as per your doctor's recommendations. Without some sort of exercise, treatment may be ineffective.

---

*To rid canned sardines of most of their salt, rinse under running water 30 to 60 seconds (never more, or you will wash away most nutrients).

**Since the findings that L-carnitine may be helpful in the prevention and treatment of heart disease are new, no official dosage has been established; you may want to consult your physician before using it.

†Do not use EPA omega-3 capsules if you are on aspirin therapy.

LIFESTYLE CONSIDERATIONS

Anger, rage, guilt, and other negative emotions raise blood pressure, elevate cholesterol, and may prove to be the most pervasive cause of most types of heart disease. See the Stress Plan. Quit smoking as well, since cigarette smoking does all of the above, too.

Herpes Plan

IDENTIFICATION AND CAUSES

The herpes virus is an opportunistic viral infection which can get inside of anyone at any age; once the virus enters the body it remains there for life, though if our immunity is strong we may never know it. The herpes may lay dormant in nerve cells, sometimes for years, waiting for a weakening of immunity so that they can create another infection. There are three strains of herpes viruses to worry about. Herpes simplex-I is marked by the presence of the common cold sore; herpes simplex-II is a sexually transmitted disease; and herpes zoster, also known as shingles, is a viral infection of nerves.

Herpes simplex-I is contagious and may be passed through kissing or sharing a toothbrush, glass, or eating utensil. Herpes simplex-II is transmitted through sexual contact and is less dormant than herpes simplex-I; recent studies show that the virus is most likely to engage in re-activity as the result of stress and other emotional causes, other infections, fevers, the use of certain drugs, alcohol, caffeine, excessive refined sugar; even drinking chlorine and other chemicals from tap water can awaken herpes simplex-II. Herpes zoster infections are most commonly caused by an old chicken pox virus that never entirely went away. Herpes zoster (street name: shingles) can be reinduced by stress, fatigue, diabetes, hidden infections, even cancer, as well as excess refined sugar, overall poor diet, alcohol, and other immune-lowering factors. It most commonly produces blisters at the nerve endings of the skin but can occur anywhere on the bodies of persons at any age, regardless of whether they ever had chicken pox; in fact many people infected with the chicken pox virus develop herpes rather than chicken pox.

SYMPTOMS

Herpes simplex (I and II) usually starts with a tingling and numbness, which turns into painful watery, often bubbling, legions, as well as discharge, blistering, and itching. Herpes zoster usually causes severe pain and itching of skin, or pain in nerves called postherpetic neuritis. Any of these symptoms requires immediate medical attention.

TREATMENT

In my own practice I have used lithium cream and ice to treat herpes with some success. I have also seen results from the prescription medication Acyclovir. You may want to discuss these approaches with your doctor. For shingles I have seen success from extra B-complex and megadoses of vitamin C, beta carotene, and L-Lysine. For active lesions, injections of 1000 micrograms per day of B-12 for one to three weeks, plus 50 milligrams per day of zinc, may help, so you may want to discuss this with your physician. There is no known cure for herpes, but the virus can be put permanently to rest through the fortification of the immune system. Pain may be relieved with antidepressants.

ANTI-HERPES DIET

Coffee, sugar, alcohol, chorinated drinking water, and drugs will worsen a herpes condition, so make an extra effort to eliminate these toxins from your body. Foods containing the amino acid arginine may also exacerbate herpes; these foods include peanuts and most other nuts, chocolate, seeds, and beans. Tap water should be filtered or avoided in favor of good quality bottled water. There are also some positive steps for treating and preventing the recurrence of the herpes virus. Foods containing lysine have been found to help, as have fish containing EPA omega-3.

REJUVENATION FOODS TO EMPHASIZE

High-lysine foods

Fish (especially all EPA-containing fish—see the Rejuvenation Diet), poultry, brewer's yeast, nonfat milk and nonfat yogurt, egg whites, white meat chicken, white meat turkey.

Oils

One tablespoon per day of borage (canola or rapeseed) oil, hybrid safflower oil, or sunflower seed oil (preferably on salad).

SUPPLEMENTS INCREASED FROM REGULAR REJUVENATION INSURANCE

For herpes simplex I and II

Beta carotene	50,000 IUs daily while lesions persist, then down to 25,000 IUs daily
B-complex	100 to 150 mgs daily
Vitamin C	As much as can be tolerated without diarrhea
Vitamin E	800 IUs daily
Zinc	30 mgs (zinc picolinate) daily
EPA tablets	300 mgs (in 1000-mg base), three times a day
L-lysine*	1200 mgs daily

For herpes zoster (shingles)

Beta carotene	50,000 IUs daily for three weeks, then down to 25,000 IUs daily
B-complex	200 mgs daily
Vitamin C	8 to 10 grams daily
Vitamin D	800 mgs daily
Calcium	1500 mgs daily
Magnesium	750 mgs daily
EPA omega-3	300 mgs (in 1000-mg base), three capsules per day

*L-lysine can elevate cholesterol so must be watched closely by your doctor.

THE EXERCISE FACTOR

Exercise is vital to the suppression of the herpes virus, as it reduces stress and raises immunity.

LIFESTYLE CONSIDERATIONS

Adequate rest is essential to keeping herpes dormant, as are lifestyle choices relating to anger, stress, depression, and the other negative emotions that can lower immunity and instigate a recurrence of herpes lesions.

High Blood Pressure Plan

IDENTIFICATION AND CAUSES

Blood pressure refers to the pressure at which the heart pushes blood throughout the body. Average normal blood pressure is around $^{120}/_{80}$. The first number refers to the pressure as the blood is being pushed throughout the body. This is called the systolic pressure. The second number is the diastolic pressure measuring the resting phase of the heartbeat; this shows how much force the blood still exerts even when the heart is not pumping. This is the friction or pressure the body pushes back against the flow of blood within it. Blood pressure anywhere below $^{145}/_{85}$ is still considered normal, but once it reaches or exceeds $^{145}/_{85}$, blood pressure is too high and should be dealt with.

High blood pressure—also known as hypertension—affects about 35 million Americans, people of all ages, but is most common in those over forty. There may be a hereditary factor involved, but some people with a family history of hypertension never develop it, and others with no family history of high blood pressure may themselves develop a severe problem due to other factors. Most cases of hypertension, in fact, are called "essential" hypertension because the cause or causes are unknown. But there are many potential reasons for blood pressure to rise.

Excess salt in the diet and activation of certain hormones, both of which cause the retention of water in the blood stream, increases the amount of fluid the heart must pump throughout the body, thus increasing the pressure it must use to accomplish this. Caffeine, alcohol, and excess sugar can also bring on hypertension. Excess body weight and cholesterol in the blood also make the heart work harder. Emotional stress and tension can cause spasms of the blood vessels, restricting the flow of blood and raising blood pressure. Fear, anxiety, and anger can release adrenaline in the body, raising blood pressure, at least temporarily; but we now know that people with hypertension are not *necessarily* overanxious or high-strung. High blood pressure may also be the result of kidney disease, but it may equally well be "essential" hypertension, meaning it is due to, or the result of, unknown causes.

SYMPTOMS

In its later stages hypertension can cause headaches, dizzy spells, fast heartbeat, shortness of breath, nosebleeds, and hot sweats. In the most extreme cases, high blood pressure can cause kidney failure or coronary heart attack. Early hypertension, however, gives few warnings. There are a lot of people out there who have high blood pressure but don't know it. Sometimes there is an early morning headache, or unexplained dizzy spells, or heart palpitations, but all too often there are no symptoms until the illness has reached critical proportions. For this reason, frequent blood pressure checks are advisable.

TREATMENT

Most doctors prescribe medications to control high blood pressure. This is usually proper procedure, as high blood pressure is a serious matter and must be alleviated as rapidly as possibly; but I have found that in many less urgent cases a modification of diet along with exercise, weight reduction, biofeedback, and the proper frame of mind are all that are needed to bring blood pressure under control. If diet is the major cause of hypertension, diet is certainly where prevention begins, and it may very well also be the key to its treatment.

ANTI-HYPERTENSION DIET

The Rejuvenation Diet *is* an anti-hypertension diet. Reducing sodium content to 1000 milligrams per day (about half a teaspoon), for most people, eliminates water retention and the need for diuretics; but please do not replace salt with salt substitutes, excessive use of which can cause heart rhythm irregularities—sometimes life-threatening ones. Instead use real nonsodium seasonings as suggested in the Rejuvenation Diet. Reducing calories to rejuvenation levels will reduce body weight and cholesterol. Eliminating coffee and consuming alcohol in only minimal amounts may bring hypertension under control immediately. If you are more than a little overweight, see the Obesity Plan, and if your cholesterol level is dangerously high, see the Cholesterol Plan.

The foods we want to emphasize in treating hypertension are those high in potassium, magnesium, and/or linoleic acid and EPA omega-3 essential fatty acids. In recent studies, all have been found to help lower blood pressure.

REJUVENATION FOODS TO EMPHASIZE

Fresh vegetables

Asparagus, broccoli, Brussels sprouts, cabbage, cauliflower, corn on the cob, eggplant, lima beans, green peas, peppers, baked potatoes, sweet potatoes, yams, radishes, summer and winter squash.

Fresh fruits

Apples, apricots, avocados, bananas, cantaloupes, dates (not dried, no sodium), grapefruits, honeydew melons, nectarines, prunes, raisins, watermelons.

Whole grains

Bran, any whole grain cereal (unprocessed, no sodium).

Oils

Olive oil, borage (canola or rapeseed) oil, sunflower seed oil.

SUPPLEMENTS INCREASED FROM REGULAR REJUVENATION INSURANCE

Several studies on calcium supplementation along with vitamin D have shown that blood pressure can be reduced 5 to 10 percent or more in a period of a few months. L-tryptophan is now known to induce calm and reduce the body's fight-or-flight mechanisms which produce adrenaline. Other studies on vitamin C link its increase with a potential lowering of blood pressure.

Vitamin C	10,000 mgs daily (or to tolerance)
Calcium	1 to 2 grams daily
EPA omega-3	5 to 10 grams daily
L-tryptophan	500 mgs, four times a day (taken on empty stomach)

THE EXERCISE FACTOR

Another reason to put on your walking shoes: Rigorous daily activity is crucial in bringing blood pressure under control. Besides burning calories, fat, and cholesterol, daily exercise increases circulation and dilates blood vessels, reducing blood pressure. If you have hypertension, however, it is advisable that you exercise under the guidance of your physician.

LIFESTYLE CONSIDERATIONS

Another reason to quit smoking: Smoking constricts the arterioles and immediately elevates blood pressure. Nicotine makes the heart beat faster, increasing its need for oxygen, and the carbon monoxide from the tobacco smoke reduces oxygen in the blood stream. Hypertension may also be your body's way of telling you to stop living in constant anger, anxiety, and stress. A recent study found that hostility alone significantly raised blood pressure. Depression was a not-too-distant second, followed by many other negative emotions. See Chapter 6 and the Stress Plan.

High Cholesterol Plan

IDENTIFICATION AND CAUSES

Cholesterol is a substance necessary to our bodies; it aids in the manufacture of all of our hormones and bile salts, and in digestion. Too much cholesterol, however, can be deadly. High cholesterol is a major health problem.

While an absolute ceiling for safe cholesterol has yet to be agreed upon, my own medical experience tells me that any amount of cholesterol above 180 milligrams per CC of blood analyzed is too high, dangerously too high. Our LDL, or low density lipoproteins (the "bad guy" cholesterol), should not exceed 90, and our HDL, or high-density lipoproteins (the "good guy" cholesterol), should not fall below 45, and preferably should be above 60.

The main cause of elevated cholesterol is the consumption of animal fats. Animal fats *are* cholesterol. One egg yolk contains about as much cholesterol as anyone should consume in an entire day. Two eggs sunny-side up with bacon is enough for the week. It is not hard, adhering to the classic American diet, to end up with high cholesterol and possible heart disease. But there are other saturated fats, such as whole milk, cheese, tropical oils (palm kernel and coconut), and any hydrogenated oil, which are metabolized into cholesterol inside the body and thus are just as deadly. A recent study, in fact, discovered some vegetarians with high cholesterol blood levels and arteriosclerosis just from eating excessive quantities of cheese. Excess refined sugars and refined carbohydrates can also be metabolized into cholesterol, as explained in the Rejuvenation Diet. No one knows why, but it is now established that cigarette smoking also raises cholesterol, as do alcohol and many drugs, a sedentary life, a stressful life, high blood pressure, and a number of other illnesses. In some people, genetic programming predisposes the body to manufacture an overabundance of cholesterol.

SYMPTOMS

There are no noticeable early symptoms of high cholesterol, and the latter symptoms are the products of high cholesterol such as heart attack and stroke. A serum cholesterol test should therefore be standard once a year for anyone over forty who plans to live another forty or sixty years (or anyone at any age, including your children), unless you presently have or have had abnormally high cholesterol, in which case it should be monitored at least every four to six months.

TREATMENT

There are a number of prescriptive medications available for lowering cholesterol. They all have potential side effects and are unnecessary except in emergency situations where there is no time to allow a change in diet and lifestyle to cure the problem. If your cholesterol is at such a dangerous level that your doctor believes medications are necessary, make sure to evaluate the potential side effects, discuss alternatives, and find out how long you will need the drug, provided you change diet and lifestyle. If your cholesterol is not at such a fatal level, I urge you to start exercising and to follow the Rejuvenation Diet, along with the following additional tips.

ANTI-HIGH-CHOLESTEROL DIET

The foods to avoid are obvious but still worth repeating. The major culprit is, of course, saturated fats. Avoid all animal fats, whole dairy, egg yolks (the whites of the egg when cooked are a good fat-free protein, whereas one egg *yolk* contains your maximum safe amount of cholesterol for an entire day!), and all tropical oils, such as palm kernel and coconut oil. Even if a label says "all vegetable oils," they may still be saturated. Anything partially hydrogenated is a saturated fat; and this means any oil, even olive oil, if heated, is no longer a safe oil.

Frying of any kind is unadvisable for anyone with high cholesterol or for anyone aiming at 180 milligrams or less of blood cholesterol. Occasional quick stir-frying, once you have cholesterol under control, may be safe, but do not think it is cholesterol-free.

In avoiding saturated fats, we must eliminate virtually all bakery products, even crackers and frozen breaded chicken and fish, which are all made with lard. (The crackers can easily be replaced with unsalted rice cakes.) Now we also have another good reason to avoid refined sugars and refined carbohydrates.

Since the Rejuvenation Diet is a low-fat, high-fiber, high-nutrient-density diet, it is already an anti-cholesterol diet. However, if your cholesterol is already at a dangerous level, you may wish to increase your fiber intake to 30 to 35 grams of fiber per every 1000 calories of food. Water-soluble fiber such as oat bran absorbs cholesterol in the blood, and water-insoluble wheat bran sweeps cholesterol out of the colon. One cup (uncooked) of oat bran per day, in fact, has been reported to lower cholesterol by as much as 20 percent. Another recent study found that losing weight alone, even if no other measures were taken, had an impact on lowering cholesterol.

In cutting out eggs and red meats, we must make sure to get enough protein. The best low-fat way to do this is with fish, soybean products, beans, and all other legumes.

In addition, there are other rejuvenation foods you may wish to emphasize, based on the latest information on the nutrition/cholesterol-lowering connection. Niacin, B-6, vitamin C, vitamin E, biotin, choline, folic acid, inositol, chromium, magnesium, manganese, potassium, vanadium, and zinc have, in various studies, all been found helpful in lowering serum cholesterol. What follows is a list of those foods most nutrient-dense in those elements; also, additional supplement insurance dosages of these vitamins and minerals.

Other research implicates omega-3 and all linoleic precursor acids as lowering LDL cholesterol without lowering good guy HDL cholesterol. In addition, I have listed the best possible fiber sources.

REJUVENATION FOODS TO EMPHASIZE

Vegetables

All leafy greens (especially turnips), dark greens (especially broccoli and Brussels sprouts), cauliflower, beets, cabbage, mushrooms, celery, garlic, onions, potatoes.

Legumes

All.

Fruits

Pears and apples (with skins), bananas, citrus fruits (uncooked), pineapples, dates, figs, apricots, kiwis, melons, all berries (especially strawberries and blackberries).

Fish

All—especially those high in EPA omega-3. See list, Rejuvenation Diet.

Other

Black pepper, brown rice, wild rice, brewer's yeast, sunflower seeds.

Oils

Olive oil, borage (canola or rapeseed) oil, hybrid safflower oil.

Water-soluble fiber

Oat bran, pectin—best found in apples and pears.

Water-insoluble fiber

Wheat bran, apples, pears, cabbage, cauliflower, root vegetables, green vegetables, pinto beans, navy beans, dried split peas.

SUPPLEMENTS INCREASED FROM REGULAR REJUVENATION INSURANCE

Vitamin C	1000 mgs, twice a day
Lecithin	1 tbsp daily
EPA omega-3	300 mgs (in 1000-mg base), one capsule per day
Niacin*	100 mgs, three times a day
Activated charcoal**	8 grams, twice a day

THE EXERCISE FACTOR

There is now a clear link between exercise and the raising of "good guy" HDL cholesterol, the lowering of "bad guy" LDL cholesterol, and the lowering of overall cholesterol.

LIFESTYLE CONSIDERATIONS

All dietary measures and the most faithful commitment to daily exercise may not lower cholesterol one milligram if stress and other negative emotions continue to run amok. See the Stress Plan.

Hyperthyroidism Plan

IDENTIFICATION AND CAUSES

Hyperthyroidism is a condition of excess thyroid hormone in the body because of excess production by the thyroid gland. Its cause is still unknown, but it is becoming increasingly apparent that this disorder, once thought to be a problem primarily of

---

*Niacin should not be used by anyone with gout, liver disease, or non–insulin-dependent diabetes. Others who have never before taken a niacin supplement may experience hyperventilation, rashes, flushes, or rapid heart rate. If so, decrease the dosage to 25 milligrams daily and increase slowly (25 milligrams per day per week) until you reach the recommended dosage.

**The link between activated charcoal and the lowering of cholesterol is a very recent finding but the potential implications are major: up to 40 percent lowering of LDL cholesterol and up to 8 percent increase in HDL. Moreover, there are no known side effects; you may want to discuss this with your doctor.

younger people, is just as likely to occur in someone over forty and is often preceded by a major bout with stress.

SYMPTOMS

When excess thyroid is produced, metabolism increases to an abnormally high rate and various organ systems enter "overdrive." This can cause weight loss and nutritional deficiencies; muscle tissue can be wasted and protein lost. Other symptoms are fatigue, weakness, irritability, anxiety and nervousness, insomnia, mood swings, intolerance to heat, rapid pulse, heart irregularities, high blood pressure, and shortness of breath; if the condition is not identified and treated within several months, rapid aging and deterioration result. Any of these symptoms present should be checked out immediately, as medical treatment is needed to bring this condition under control.

TREATMENT

Most doctors use isotope or prescriptive therapy, which should be followed according to their recommendations. There are also dietary considerations that you might want to bring to your doctor's attention.

ANTI-HYPERTHYROIDISM DIET

Caffeine, alcohol, and tobacco all can make a hyperthyroid condition worse, increasing metabolism and further depleting the body's nutrients. Avoid these substances.

In order to rebuild the body from a hyperthyroid condition, you need to double the recommended protein for the Rejuvenation Diet, although you still want to obtain it from low-fat, low-sodium, unprocessed sources, especially nonfat dairy, plant sources, and deep-water fish. If severely underweight you will want to increase caloric consumption temporarily, but again, get these calories through lean proteins and complex carbohydrates.

There are additional supplements that will also aid in rebuilding the body. Ask your physician to consider them.

SUPPLEMENTS INCREASED FROM REGULAR REJUVENATION INSURANCE

Beta carotene	50,000 IUs daily
B-complex	150 mgs daily
Thiamin	200 mgs daily
Choline	1000 mgs daily
EPA capsules	300 mgs (in 1000-mg base), three times a day

THE EXERCISE FACTOR

See Chapter 5.

LIFESTYLE CONSIDERATIONS

See Chapter 6.

Hypothyroidism Plan

IDENTIFICATION AND CAUSE

Hypothyroidism is a deficiency of the thyroid hormone in our body as a result of a lack of thyroid production or an inability to use the hormone. Until recently it was believed to be of concern only to young people, but it is now increasingly common in people over forty because of our atmospheric contamination of iodine from atomic energy testing of the past forty years, as well as increased iodine making its way into our food supply. Iodine, in excess, stops the thyroid gland from manufacturing the hormone. In fact, Iodine used to be a prescription for *hyper*thyroidism. Hypothyroidism can also be induced by stress and trauma, as in surgery. It is often either undiagnosed in older persons or misdiagnosed as senility or aging, and must always be considered as a possible cause for the following symptoms.

SYMPTOMS

Tiredness, lethargy, fatigue, poor memory, confusion, depression, immobility, moodiness, loss of libido, tingling of hands and feet, unexplained sense of coldness, poor sleep, constipation, swelling, dry skin, itchiness, loss of hair, loss of appetite, and, more common than many people know, heart failure can all be symptomatic of hypothyroidism, and the persistence of any one or more of these symptoms warrants a doctor's attention with a thyroid hormone blood test.

TREATMENT

Treatment requires replacement hormone therapy prescribed by a physician once a positive diagnosis has been made. There are no dietary considerations beyond the Rejuvenation Diet and no additional supplements needed to treat this condition, but you must be extra careful to avoid food sources contaminated with iodine (see Recommended Reading section for toxicology books).

THE EXERCISE FACTOR

See Chapter 5.

LIFESTYLE CONSIDERATIONS

See Chapter 6.

Indigestion Plan

IDENTIFICATION AND CAUSES

Indigestion, one of the most common complaints among Americans, especially those over 40, is actually a symptom and not an illness. It is a symptom of overeating, especially refined sugars and excess fats and proteins, which causes abdominal pain. When too much food lands in the stomach at once, the stomach bloats and can shoot excess acid back up at the esophagus (as if to tell the mouth to quit eating). When the acid hits the esophagus lining it can feel like the early symptoms of a heart attack; hence the name "heartburn." Other causes of indigestion are gastric ulcers, food allergies, lack of proper fiber, lack of proper fluids, especially water, and too much alcohol and/or coffee.

SYMPTOMS

Since indigestion is actually a symptom itself, I will only add that it can manifest as a burning sensation in the chest or abdomen, along with a pressure sensation. It is often accompanied by gas pains, constipation, and irritable bowel syndrome.

TREATMENT

In cases where indigestion can be linked to a bout with overeating or excessive drinking, medical treatment is probably not needed. Antacids may temporarily relieve the discomfort, though I do not recommend their use more than very occasionally, because not only are many of them high in sodium and contain aluminum but also because the discomfort they are relieving should be painful enough to act as a deterrent to overeating in the future.

If, however, indigestion occurs without overeating, it can be a food allergy, food poisoning, or any number of other causes, from ulcers to pancreatitis to liver disease, and should be checked by your physician.

ANTI-INDIGESTION DIET

Once the cause of indigestion can be identified, the solutions should be obvious. The Rejuvenation Diet should eliminate indigestion, unless it is being caused by a food allergy. There are no particular rejuvenation foods or supplements we need to emphasize, but if accompanying gas is a problem, see the Irritable Bowel Syndrome Plan for rejuvenation foods to avoid. If overeating is clearly the cause, thank your body for causing a discomfort that may in the long run save your life.

THE EXERCISE FACTOR

Lack of exercise can be a contributory factor in any number of stomach disorders, and thus rigorous activity can play an important role in treatment.

LIFESTYLE CONSIDERATIONS

If overeating is the cause, see the Obesity Plan. After feeding yourself you deserve to feel satisfied and well-nourished, not sick.

Irritable Bowel Syndrome Plan

IDENTIFICATION AND CAUSES

Probably the most frequent digestive complaint among men and women over forty (occurring in three times as many women than men), irritable bowel syndrome may also be the most underdiagnosed digestive illness. It is usually a chronic condition and related to inappropriate, inadequate, or malfunctioning of the muscle fiber within the colon; this means the colon dilates and distends, is sluggish and spastic, and normal harmonic contractions supposed to move food along cease, allowing excess fermentation. It may be caused by stress, allergies, excess sugars, or excess fats. In some rare cases, it can be accompanied by other gastrointestinal illnesses such as parasite disease, ileitis, or colitis.

SYMPTOMS

The most common complaints associated with this syndrome are abdominal distress or cramping, erratic frequency of bowel movement, and variation in the consistency of the stool, often alternating between constipation and diarrhea. Sometimes a combination of these symptoms, or all symptoms, may occur simultaneously, accompanied by a lump in the throat, nausea, bloating, belching, and flatulence. Sometimes passing gas temporarily relieves abdominal pain, but often it only increases the discomfort. This condition, not surprisingly, can cause weakness, fatigue, lassitude, and depression. Any or all of these symptoms, however, can also be caused by growths, tumors, or other obstructions in the intestine or colon, so a doctor's examination is necessary for accurate diagnosis. An awareness on your part of the possibility of irritable bowel syndrome can be the difference between misdiagnosis and proper diagnosis and treatment.

TREATMENT

Intestinal studies are in order, including endoscopes (which look inside with light and mirror), X rays, and a gastrointestinal (GI) workup to rule out serious disease. Beyond that, dietary measures and stress reduction are the most effective treatment available at any price.

ANTI–IRRITABLE BOWEL SYNDROME DIET

The Rejuvenation Diet will provide a good basis for the nutritional treatment of this illness, cutting out the excess saturated fats, refined sugars, and refined carbohydrates, and the barrage of processed foods that can instigate and aggravate irritated bowels. You will need to be extra careful about coffee, tea, and artificial sweeteners, especially sorbitol, which by itself can bring on this syndrome. Eating more slowly and chewing longer also play an important role. In addition, there are some rejuvenation foods to temporarily avoid, if you find that they produce gas, and some rejuvenation foods to emphasize.

REJUVENATION FOODS TO AVOID

Vegetables

Brussels sprouts, carrots, cabbage, celery, garlic, onions, baked potatoes.

Legumes

All beans, lentils.

All dairy products except nonfat yogurt.

All nuts and seeds.

REJUVENATION FOODS TO EMPHASIZE

Whole grains

Brown rice, wheat or oat bran (three tablespoons daily), unprocessed bran cereal (three to six ounces daily).

Fresh vegetables

All not listed to avoid; they should be steamed.

Fresh fruits

Any (three per day), especially dried or fresh figs.

Legumes

Soybean.

Dairy

Nonfat yogurt.

Other

Herb teas (especially peppermint), or one cup of hot water with one tablespoon blackstrap molasses; two to four tablespoons daily of a soy-based acidophilus liquid.

THE EXERCISE FACTOR

The more the better; rigorous activity is vital to restoring colon function to normal.

LIFESTYLE CONSIDERATIONS

See the Stress Plan.

Kidney Stone Plan

IDENTIFICATION AND CAUSES

When an excess of certain minerals—primarily phosphates, oxylates, calcium, and urates—are present in excess at any given time in either kidney, or if the kidneys for some reason are unable to metabolize such minerals, a crystal is formed, known as a kidney stone. People who drink large quantities of carbonated sugared colas, which are loaded with phosphates, are more prone to kidney stones. A vitamin B-6 deficiency can cause oxylates to form excessively, forming kidney stones. Gout, generally a genetically predisposed disease characterized by high uric acid levels in the blood, can also cause kidney stones. High-calcium waste produced by a hyperthyroid disease is another possible cause. Excess protein, caffeine, and alcohol may produce kidney stones; a recent report has also linked high sucrose consumption to this condition. A magnesium deficiency can unbalance kidney functions, thus also causing the formation of kidney stones. The latest estimates indicate that about 5 percent of all Americans have a kidney stone at any given time.

SYMPTOMS

As the stone grows in size, it can obstruct the flow of urine, causing sharp and/or constant pain. If the stone decides to come down the urinary tract, it will, of course, cause great discomfort as it passes out. Other acute pain associated with these crystals can occur in the back, on either side, depending on which kidney the stone is lodged in. Or there may be pain in the groin, or in men, testicular pain. If you have any reason to suspect that you may have a kidney stone, see your doctor. While kidney stones can sometimes pass safely—if not painlessly—out of the urethra, they may remain and obstruct urination, thus causing blood in the urine and serious injury to the kidney.

TREATMENT

Once your physician has determined the presence of a kidney stone, forcing fluids (that is, making you drink lots of water if you do not already do so) may help you pass the stone. If that does not work, a surgical technique may be necessary for its safe removal. The new use of sound waves to fracture kidney stones may help to prevent surgery.

ANTI–KIDNEY STONE DIET

Aside from avoiding high-phosphorus soft drinks, caffeine, excess alcohol, and excess protein, there are no foods to further emphasize. I do, however, prescribe ten to fourteen glasses of *filtered* water per day; the chlorine found in most tap water causes stones in some people. Since kidney stones may be caused by deficiencies in either vitamin B-6 or magnesium, we want to increase those supplemental levels. Others, who do not process calcium properly, may need to reduce dietary calcium. Increasing magnesium may enable us to maintain a proper calcium intake, not to exceed 1500 milligrams daily.

SUPPLEMENTS INCREASED FROM REGULAR REJUVENATION INSURANCE

Vitamin B-6	100 mgs daily
Magnesium	1000 mgs daily

THE EXERCISE FACTOR

See Chapter 5.

LIFESTYLE CONSIDERATIONS

See Chapter 6.

Lower Back Pain Plan

IDENTIFICATION AND CAUSES

Lower back pain is a most ubiquitous illness, suffered by nearly 80 percent of all people at least once during their lives. Of that 80 percent, 20 percent are chronic.

The most common cause is a muscle tendon strain related to poor position, posture, some mechanical stretch or pull, or just spending too many hours each day in a poorly designed automobile seat, desk chair, or sagging mattress. Chronic lower back pain is usually the consequence of obesity, lack of exercise, poor muscle tone, poor posture, menstruation, and, more often than was previously believed, stress. Recent findings, however, point to another potentially common cause: the consumption of excess polyunsaturated oils. These so-called "safe" oils ("safe" because they don't raise cholesterol) will in excess be converted by the body into large quantities of arachidonic acid, which in quantities beyond the body's needs is a causative agent in muscle aches of all kinds, including lower back pains. In some cases, of course, the cause is of a more serious nature, such as a sprained disc, a local lesion, muscle spasms, tumors, fractures, arthritis, or osteoporosis, so a physician is always needed to make a proper diagnosis.

SYMPTOMS

There is no question: you know when you have lower back pain. The pain can be sharp and very localized, or it can be general and move about the back. Stiffness is often present, and in order to compensate for the lower back pain, the body's realignment can often cause neck and other muscle and joint pain.

TREATMENT

Your physician's diagnosis, possibly done with X rays and CT and MRI scans, will determine the kind of treatment. Often all that is needed is heat and bed rest on a firm mattress, or a new desk chair or an added support to a car seat. A regular exercise program and weight loss (see the Obesity Plan) is often the answer.

Some common medical treatments include the medicine colchicine, a two-hundred-year-old drug and still one of the best aids for chronic disc and back pain. Muscle-relaxant drugs may be helpful, as may anti-inflammatory medications. Any drug, however, causes side effects and must be considered with that in mind, and reevaluated often. Specific back exercises may be the most helpful tool, and they have no known side effects. Make sure your back specialist prescribes thirty minutes to an hour's worth of these per day.

ANTI-LOWER BACK PAIN DIET

Since excess polyunsaturates may be the cause—or part of the cause—of your lower back pain, I suggest that you eliminate (or virtually eliminate) their use, replacing them with minimal quantities of monounsaturates such as olive oil, borage (canola or rapeseed) oil. Otherwise adhere to the Rejuvenation Diet guidelines, though there are supplemental increases that may help.

SUPPLEMENTS INCREASED FROM REGULAR REJUVENATION INSURANCE

B-complex	150 mgs daily
Thiamin	100 mgs daily
Calcium	1500 mgs daily
Magnesium*	1000 mgs daily
EPA omega-3**	300 mgs (in 1000-mg base), one capsule three times a day
L-tryptophan	400 mgs, four times a day

THE EXERCISE FACTOR

In addition to specific back exercises, walking forty minutes to an hour is essential to strengthening the back muscles, making them more flexible and durable. Since this kind of activity is recommended for about one hundred other health reasons and is a major longevity factor, your lower back pain may turn out to be a key factor in extending your life. Hatha yoga is also a valuable tool in the treatment of lower back pain, as it not only improves musculature but helps to relieve stress and the other emotional causes. But be sure to get a trained yoga teacher and avoid hyperextending the back.

---

*Do not take this much magnesium if you have kidney disease.

**Do not take EPA if you are, for any reason, on aspirin therapy.

LIFESTYLE CONSIDERATIONS

Lower back pain for many people may come down to a self-esteem issue. "Am I worth a good firm mattress? A car or desk seat with good support? Am I important enough to deserve a free hour a day in which to exercise?" It is remarkable, and sad, what the answers are for many people. It isn't too late to change your answers. I have prescribed biofeedback and meditation for my patients whose lower back pain seems to be the result of stress. See Chapter 6 and the Stress Plan.

I have also sent patients to a good acupressurist or acupuncturist and seen impressive results, though I do not as a rule prescribe this treatment for patients who do not first express an interest.

Malabsorption Syndrome Plan

IDENTIFICATION AND CAUSES

Among the most serious and widespread stomach disorders currently seen by doctors, malabsorption is the inability to absorb nutrients consumed in food. It can be general malabsorption of all nutrients, or malabsorption of only specific nutrients. This disorder may be attributed to liver or bile tract diseases, pancreatic disorders, inflammation of the intestines (ileitis, colitis), malignancies, food allergies, and/or at least twenty-five other diseases, ranging from enzyme deficiencies to parasites to infected mucus linings. It can also be caused by lowered hydrochloric acid (HCL) production in the stomach as we age.

SYMPTOMS

The classic symptom of malabsorption syndrome is intermittent diarrhea, occurring because of the difficulty in digesting food, especially fats. Weight loss and greater stool mass are common, as are abdominal pain, constant bloating, and flatus. Calcium malabsorption can cause a decrease in bone calcium leading to easy fractures. Poor absorption of iron, folic acid, and vitamin B-12 can cause anemia, and other vitamin deficiencies—especially vitamin D—are also likely. Lack of thiamin and the other B vitamins can cause a neuritis (a nerve problem of the legs and hands), as well as water retention edema (swollen legs). Sometimes the only symptom is chronic bone pain, and in rare cases in some men, the only symptom of advanced malabsorption syndrome is impotence—the first sign of an endocrine system beginning to fail from testosterone precursors not being absorbed. If you suffer from any of the above symptoms, you and your doctor should consider malabsorption as a possible cause.

TREATMENT

Treating this syndrome begins with identifying it and determining its cause. This requires that your physician do a variety of laboratory studies. Most important are a Sudan fat stain test to measure the amount of stool fats, and a triolein test to measure the excretion of radioactive carbon dioxide in the breath (people with malabsorption tend to exhale much less carbon dioxide than do others). Once this disorder is diagnosed, it is important that your doctor find the causative disease and treat it appropriately.

When no findings indicate the cause of a malabsorption problem, malignancy should be suspected. Otherwise, food allergies may be the culprit. Often a gluten-free diet completely void of all wheat products and rich in other non-wheat grains can completely reverse the condition. Other potentially responsible foods can be eggs, soy products, chicken, or fish.

Treatment must also include the replacement of the missing nutrients in the body, sometimes with extra supplements. Since every case is different, I cannot suggest a universal malabsorption diet plan, other than to make sure your doctor determines all of your particular deficiencies. The Rejuvenation Diet along with exercise and a positive frame of mind will act as a good foundation for recovery from this condition.

Obesity Plan

IDENTIFICATION AND CAUSES

According to the generally accepted medical definition, obesity is characterized by a condition of 100 pounds or more of excess weight. More than 17 percent of all Americans fall into this category, which puts them at high risk for a myriad of physical and emotional problems, including hypertension, diabetes mellitus, gallbladder disease, diminished lung function, increased burden on the heart, depression, and general premature aging. But one does not have to be 100 pounds overweight in order to put one's health in jeopardy. For some people, 50 extra pounds can do as much damage as 150 can to others, and as far as I'm concerned this plan also speaks to people 10 pounds overweight. Recent studies at Harvard Medical School found measurable health risks from being only somewhat overweight. High blood pressure and type II diabetes are strongly associated with any amount of excess weight; in addition, bodily fat damages blood vessels and increases the risk of heart disease.

The causes of obesity are complex and highly specific to the individual. For some, simply cutting out the high-fat convenience foods, or certain appetite-stimulating or metabolic-influencing medications, will diminish the tendency to overeat. For others who are chronically overweight there may be some sort of eating disorder. (See the Addiction Plan.) Lack of exercise and a sedentary life play an equally destructive role, but are easily remedied. There are also, of course, hereditary factors contributing to obesity, but, as with most other hereditary problems, they can cease with whatever generation makes the commitment to outlive—to *far outlive*—their genes. I have seen it happen. No one ever *has* to be obese, or even overweight, anymore.

SYMPTOMS

It might seem all too obvious to mention the symptoms: 50 or 100 pounds of fat spread over a human body is hard to avoid noticing. Yet, ironically, many obese people I have encountered have not acknowledged to themselves that they are obese. They rarely look at themselves in the mirror, and when I have persuaded obese patients to face a piece of reflecting glass, most often they see nothing from the neck down. It is very painful to see themselves as they really are, but until the obese person does, there is not much chance of recovering. However, once the obese person recognizes the problem (not by being told, which usually only strengthens denial), the most important step is then taken toward recovery.

TREATMENT

Weight loss is a billion-dollar industry, offering up the latest "miracle" diet, "magic" weight loss pill (prescription and over-the-counter), predigested protein powder, and radical medical approaches—from injecting cow urine to stapling stomachs to mutilating the intestinal tract so that food intake bypasses the stomach. Most of these approaches to weight loss not only fail to work on a long-term basis but can also create extreme health problems, from hypertension to heart disease to death. In some cases, such as hypothyroidism, medical intervention can help to restore a healthy body weight, but in most cases the answer to obesity is simple: eat less, exercise more, treat the underlying cause of the overeating.

ANTI-OBESITY DIET

The Rejuvenation Diet is the best foundation for any sane and lasting weight loss plan. There is no way an obese person can avoid losing weight if she or he reduces caloric intake to rejuvenation levels and greatly diminishes saturated fats, refined sugars and refined carbohydrates, and salt. We must be extra careful of salt while losing weight; excess sodium can stimulate the appetite, as can refined sugars, many artificial sweeteners, and caffeine (beware of sodium and caffeine in over-the-counter medications).

Depending on how much weight you need to lose, or at what stage you are in weight loss, you may find that you need to temporarily cut calories to 20 percent under suggested rejuvenation levels until you reach the desired weight. In prescribing weight-loss diets to my patients I try not to force them to measure food, but rather to become accustomed to eating in moderate amounts. Experience tells me that if a person wants to overeat and you restrict him or her to two pieces of chicken, then invariably the two pieces of chicken will be the left half and the right half. Once the commitment to eat for longevity is made, however, moderation is not hard to come by. When the recipe says two servings, eat half of what's there. Restaurant portions are usually at least a good indication of the maximum boundaries of moderation. By eating high-fiber, low-fat, low-refined–carbohydrate foods and by chewing slowly, eating should produce a feeling of fullness and send the correct message from stomach to brain that feeding time is over.

I also do not believe in limiting one's selection of fruits and vegetables. Though some fruits may contain more calories than others, if weight loss is going to be part of a lifestyle it is best if it avoids seeming like deprivation; and the number of calories in a banana as opposed to a grapefruit are not likely to keep us from overcoming obesity, whereas the feeling of deprivation very well might.

With that in mind, there are certain rejuvenation foods you may wish to emphasize. Jalapeño peppers, for those who can tolerate them, have been found to increase the body's metabolism, increasing the amount of calories used by up to 25 percent; other foods, such as bananas, berries, kiwis, and figs, even in small amounts, seem to help satisfy the craving for sweets without causing the onset of compulsive eating, and in general seem to help satisfy the appetite of people who are not used to ever feeling hungry.

REJUVENATION FOODS TO EMPHASIZE

Fresh fruits

All; about three per day. And try a frozen banana as a treat.

Vegetables

Baked potatoes, sweet potatoes, yams, raw carrots, banana squash, Jalapeño peppers.

Whole grains

Home-popped (unbuttered, unsalted) popcorn, puffed wheat, puffed rice, kasha (buckwheat groats).

Dairy

Nonfat milk, nonfat yogurt.

Others

White meat turkey, sour pickle.*

SUPPLEMENTS INCREASED FROM REGULAR REJUVENATION INSURANCE

See the Addiction Plan.

THE EXERCISE FACTOR

If you are obese, you may not be ingesting excess calories; you may just be underusing them. Exercise is crucial to reversing obesity. All who come to my office looking for a way to lose weight are immediately told that without at least a forty-minute walk per day, or equivalent other exercise, they might as well not bother to change their diet. Those who have never before exercised regularly soon discover how much easier losing weight is if they modify their eating along with a program of rigorous activity.

LIFESTYLE CONSIDERATIONS

Do not skip meals! Skipping meals usually leads to the hunger—and rationalization—that causes you to eat twice as much

*The sour pickle is an emergency food and should be used only in cases where a hot fudge sundae or equivalent seems inevitable. While the pickle is high in salt, it may be valuable in eradicating the craving for sweets (which often contain as much salt, plus refined sugar and saturated fat).

at the next meal. Avoid the feeling of deprivation. Do not focus on the foods you are choosing not to eat but on the extra life you are going to be able to live. As you lose weight and gain self-esteem, don't ever forget how lousy you felt before. Sometimes that reminder alone is all one needs to maintain.

Osteoporosis Plan

IDENTIFICATION AND CAUSES

One of the most exciting pieces of recent medical information is the realization that this painful and debilitating disease might not be an inevitability of aging.

Osteoporosis is simply decalcification of the bones, seen in people over forty, more often women. Some theories about this illness have concluded that it is caused by lack of calcium in the diet, and point to countless studies of Americans, especially women, who consume on the average 600 to 800 milligrams (half of what they need) per day. Further investigation indicates that much of the cause may begin early in a woman's life, when she stops drinking milk in favor of soda pop, which is loaded with calcium-depleting phosphorus, and as women (even when they are still girls) start exercising less or begin eating too much protein. Other more recent studies have indicated that a deficiency in either magnesium or manganese can by itself cause osteoporosis, even for people who consume 150 percent of their daily needed calcium. Alcohol abuse, cigarette smoking, and long-term use of corticosteroid drugs have also recently been linked to increased risk of osteoporosis. Others still believe the reason so many women develop osteoporosis is from loss of estrogen hormone as they enter menopause, since estrogen deficiency prevents utilization of calcium in the bones. Still others maintain that the primary cause for the increase in cases of osteoporosis is that more and more people are living longer, and that it is an inevitability of old age. I do not believe that at all.

SYMPTOMS

Backaches, bone aches, and muscle aches that are not the result of injury or strenuous exercise are all early symptoms of osteoporosis. This pain may be very similar to the pain of arthritis, and thus must be diagnosed by a physician. As the disease progresses, the skeletal structure can become twisted in a condition known as "dowager's hump," which can actually shorten us. Bones become increasingly brittle until they can easily fracture.

TREATMENT

Those who believe lack of estrogen to be the primary cause of osteoporosis insist that hormone therapy is essential, maintaining that without estrogen and progesterone there is no way to prevent or treat this disease. These hormones, however, are controversial and may be dangerous. There is evidence that exogenous sources of estrogen and other hormones may cause blood clots, heart attacks, and cancer. Recent studies, however, have confirmed my longtime suspicion that the treatment and prevention of osteoporosis are synonymous. Even after menopause, all that is necessary for good healthy bone density is a sufficient intake of vitamin D, calcium, magnesium, and manganese, coupled with the right kind of exercise. One study found that without estrogen therapy, bone density was significantly improved if these dietary measures were undertaken. Another recent study found that a natural hormone in salmon (calcitonin) may, without the side effects of exogenous hormones such as estrogens, be another effective tool in wiping out this crippling illness.

ANTI-OSTEOPOROSIS DIET

The Rejuvenation Diet is already an anti-osteoporosis diet, with its nutrient-dense foods, many of them high in vitamin D, calcium, magnesium, and manganese. It also eliminates coffee and other unhealthy foods and nonfoods that deplete these important vitamins and minerals. If, however, you already have osteoporosis, you may wish to further emphasize those rejuvenation foods highest in vitamin D, calcium, magnesium, and manganese; and you also may wish to get extra vitamin D from the most plentiful source: sunlight. If sufficient levels of these key nutrients seem ineffective, if a radiologist still finds bone density to be low, it may be a sign that you suffer from malabsorption syndrome. (See the Malabsorption Syndrome Plan.) We now also know that a hormone found naturally in salmon, known as salmon calcitonin, may, along with our recommended daily dosage of calcium and other key minerals, improve bone density by up to 13 percent. So you should certainly consider focusing your protein needs on this deep-water fish, which we already know to be one of our best foods.

REJUVENATION FOODS TO EMPHASIZE

For calcium

All nonfat dairy, sardines, salmon, all shellfish, blackstrap molasses, whole grains, dark green vegetables, root vegetables (especially carrots), sesame seeds.

For vitamin D

All nonfat dairy.

For magnesium

Wheat germ and other whole grains, blackstrap molasses, soy beans, and all fish, nuts, and seeds.

*For manganese**

Whole grains, dark green vegetables, legumes, bananas, pineapples.

For salmon calcitonin

Fresh, delicious salmon.

---

*For some reason, many people have difficulty absorbing manganese from their food, so a supplemental dosage may be essential no matter how much we consume (see next section).

SUPPLEMENTS INCREASED FROM REGULAR REJUVENATION INSURANCE

Vitamin D	400 IUs daily
Calcium	1200 to 1500 mgs daily
Magnesium	1000 mgs daily
Manganese	10 mgs daily

THE EXERCISE FACTOR

Exercising to prevent and/or treat osteoporosis has a different set of guidelines from a regular aerobic or relaxation-type exercise program, though many of the same exercises will work for two or all three criteria. The kind of exercise needed to deal with osteoporosis is the *weight-bearing* kind, which puts stress on the long bones—the back bone, pelvic bone, hip and leg bones. These include walking, jogging, and climbing stairs; they do *not* include swimming, bike riding, rowing, or any other movement that does not pit us against gravity. Studies have also found that this kind of weight-bearing exercise must be done for a minimum of fifty-five minutes, at least three times per week, in order to prevent or treat osteoporosis.

Even if you have advanced osteoporosis, hurry up and start exercising along with our diet and supplement program. It isn't too late!

LIFESTYLE CONSIDERATIONS

See Chapter 6.

Chronic Pain Plan

IDENTIFICATION AND CAUSES

Almost every day we doctors see a large number of people who complain of pain in any number of specific or general parts of the body—or of overall achiness—but upon examination show no symptoms to indicate what is causing the pain. They are always in pain and cannot tell you why. These people do not have arthritis or osteoporosis or any other bone or muscle disorder; they do not suffer from food allergies. The cause of their pain is almost always a psychological one, coupled with underused muscles and joints.

SYMPTOMS

By the time I see him or her, the chronic pain complainer is usually taking multiple medications prescribed by multiple doctors, none of whom really knew what they were treating. These people often spend much of their time in bed, have little or no joy in life, and are often either unemployed or do work that doesn't call upon their true skills. They may have very few personal relationships and are both anxious and depressed, as well as full of anger and frustration that no doctor has yet been able to cure their pain. They are known to physicians as "doctor shoppers," always blaming their pain on the last doctor who failed to cure them. Their pain often becomes a manipulative tool, not only for them but for other members of the family in various ways, very similar to the manner in which many families respond to an alcoholic member.

TREATMENT

Any physician who continues to prescribe medication for a chronic pain complainer is doing that patient a severe disservice. The only hope for treatment is to reduce drugs, habitual use of which may induce physical disorder by themselves, and to begin some form of behavior modification, usually through therapy. An increase in activity is essential. Biofeedback may do wonders to put such a detached person in touch with his or her body, and family therapy as well as group therapy may be needed.

ANTI–CHRONIC PAIN DIET

Just as the chronic pain sufferer must lose the attitude that there is a pill for every ill, he or she must not start believing that there is a food or a vitamin capsule to fix what is a psychological problem. There are, therefore, no additional foods or supplements to emphasize.

The Rejuvenation Diet by itself, however, will help to improve general health, enabling the chronic pain sufferer to see that his or her problem is not physical. By often making a person look better, the Rejuvenation Diet may also help to elevate self-worth, something the common pain complainer is desperately lacking.

THE EXERCISE FACTOR

Activity is imperative, even if it begins only with a walk to the corner three times a day. Lack of participation by the chronic pain complainer in his or her own treatment will render it useless. At least in the beginning, family members must often help by getting the chronic pain complainer out of bed and by no longer literally pampering him or her to death.

LIFESTYLE CONSIDERATIONS

Lifestyle is everything. Chronic pain is very much a self-esteem issue. For most who suffer from it, chronic pain is an illness that they must *choose* to give up, or it will never go away.

Psoriasis Plan

IDENTIFICATION AND CAUSE

By far the most common condition prompting men and women over forty to see a dermatologist, psoriasis is a progressive skin disorder caused by the overgrowth of surface skin. Prostaglandins may be in the link of causes, but no one is really sure. Heredity and stress are certainly major contributing factors; stress is an especially significant cause of flare-ups of psoriasis.

SYMPTOMS

The small or large lesions are most often patchy, red and whitish, scaly, circular, most frequently occurring on the legs, arms, lower back, scalp, and ears. Sometimes they are itchy, sometimes not, but they are almost always unsightly and potentially embarrassing.

TREATMENT

Doctors often prescribe ultraviolet light, backyard sunshine, or laboratory-based PUVA light treatment. One recent report cited the sun rays at the Dead Sea beaches in Israel as having a miraculous curative effect on psoriasis. But this is not of much use to those of you who aren't planning to move to the Middle East, and over extended periods of time, all such ultraviolet therapy may increase the risk of skin cancer and thus should not be conducted in excess—and for those at high risk for skin cancer, not at all. There are also a variety of tar-based and cortisone-based creams and ointments available, which may or may not work to relieve the symptoms. There is no official cure for psoriasis, but there are some nutritional measures we can take that may keep it in remission for the rest of our lives.

ANTI-PSORIASIS DIET

Since animal fats can increase the severity of this condition in some people, we want to be extra careful to avoid these; this includes the fat of all poultry, such as chicken skin. On the positive side, essential fatty acids seem to be remarkably helpful in bringing psoriasis under control in some patients. Since stress often worsens this condition, also see the Stress Plan for additional dietary and supplementation recommendations.

REJUVENATION FOODS TO EMPHASIZE

Fish

Mackerel, herring, sardines, salmon.

Whole grains

Wheat germ.

Oils

Olive oil, borage (canola or rapeseed) oil, sunflower seed oil, fish oil.

SUPPLEMENTS INCREASED FROM REGULAR REJUVENATION INSURANCE

Beta carotene	50,000 IUs daily for the first three weeks; 25,000 IUs daily thereafter
Vitamin C	up to 4000 mgs daily (as tolerated)
Vitamin E*	400 IUs daily for the first month; 800 IUs daily for second month; 1200 IUs daily for third month
EPA omega-3**	one to six daily (300 mgs in 1000-mg base)
Lecithin	two tbsps daily
Olive oil	one tbsp daily (unless you are consuming it as part of diet)

THE EXERCISE FACTOR

Do not allow skin discomfort to prevent you from taking care of the rest of your health. Exercise, if it helps reduce stress, may help diminish the symptoms of psoriasis.

LIFESTYLE CONSIDERATIONS

Since stress often worsens psoriasis (not to mention other skin disorders), see the Stress Plan. Also, avoid artificial fabrics and wool; use only cotton clothing to cover psoriasis lesions.

Stress Plan

IDENTIFICATION AND CAUSES

Scientifically speaking, stress is any physical or mental stimulus—such as fear, pain, or exhilaration—that disturbs or inter-

*Do not use vitamin E in these high doses if you have high blood pressure.

**Do not take EPA while taking aspirin and do not take more than one EPA tablet while on anticoagulents prescribed by a physician.

feres with the normal physiological equilibrium of an organism. I mention this because stress has become something of a buzzword, with many vague meanings. Stress is not necessarily a negative phenomenon, not by any means. Clearly, there is good stress and there is bad stress. Winning the lottery would probably instigate a good kind of stress, while being visited shortly thereafter by the IRS would likely bring on the bad kind of stress. We already know from Chapter 6 that too much bad stress can contribute to virtually any medical disability and that it is perhaps the sole cause of some diseases. Recent estimates indicate that for persons over the age of forty, 50 percent to 70 percent of illness is at least related to stress.

Stress can affect our eating habits, which can also affect our health; but at the same time stress may be affected *by* our diet. Food allergies can produce very severe stress, as can certain drugs, including caffeine and alcohol. In contrast, the right kinds of foods may be able to help us relieve certain stresses. While I firmly believe that most stress is caused by—and therefore must be dealt with through—our attitudes and choices about how we live our lives, there are times in all of our lives when events beyond our control pile up and throw us into a state of "stress-surrender."

SYMPTOMS

The symptoms of stress are varied and complex. Many times they manifest as an illness—high blood pressure, arthritis, angina, high cholesterol, psoriasis, ulcers, to name a few. Hyperventilation, a rapid, shallow form of breathing often mistaken for asthma, is a common symptom of extreme stress, and is known as an anxiety attack. Often the symptoms of stress, such as fatigue, diminished intellectual insight, muscle aches and pains, headaches, itches, rashes, hives, and diarrhea, do not appear until after the stressful period is over; the body functions at its peak during the crisis, as a survival mechanism, and then breaks down once the crisis is over.

TREATMENT

Many doctors still prescribe tranquilizers, which temporarily relieve the stress reaction without in any way dealing with its cause, leading in many cases to drug dependency, increased tolerance (the need for more of the drug to get the same calming effects), and ultimately drug addiction. There is no evidence whatsoever that the artificial calm produced by these narcotics prevents stress-induced illness or in any way increases longevity; and there is great reason to believe that these drugs may, if used for extended periods of time, compromise health and decrease longevity. The only other standard medical treatment for severe stress is psychotherapy, which is a major part of the recovery of many people—unless the main cause of their stress is the ten cups of coffee and the half dozen donuts they had for breakfast. Recently it has become increasingly clear that food allergies (as well as other allergies) play a role in the onset of stress, and the allergist is becoming as important as the shrink. Even a symptom as severe as hyperventilation may be caused by cashew nuts or the formaldehyde coming off the face of the kitchen clock. Some of the most recent studies on stress may put the dietitian or nutritionist in an equally important role in treating this condition.

ANTI-STRESS DIET

Even after having eliminated all allergenic foods and substances, there will likely still be times when it is difficult for us to avoid stress; when stress, in a sense, comes looking for us. During such times it is a challenge to keep our immunity up and our health at an optimum state.

Some people, when under severe or even moderate stress, tend to eat little or nothing. This is a big mistake. Failure to consume adequate amounts of food lowers blood sugar and can set off an emergency chemical response in the body, increasing stress. Stress incurred in this way may last far longer than the initial stress. Another common but serious dietary mistake is eating refined carbohydrates for temporary sedation. The sedation is caused by the quick raising of blood sugar, but this produces an insulin response which soon lowers blood sugar below the previously low level, producing excessive flow of adrenaline, doubling or tripling the sense of stress and tension.

Following the Rejuvenation Diet will eliminate the possibility of intensifying stress through eating, and there are certain rejuvenation foods that for some people can help to diminish this kind of stress. The B-complex vitamins—thiamin, niacin, B-6, and folic acid—all play key roles in our nervous system and have started to become a part of phobic therapy. Other nutrients—to be obtained from food sources as well as supplemental insurance—that are most likely to act as natural tranquilizers for us seem to be calcium, magnesium, and the amino acid L-tryptophan. We also want to make sure we are getting extra vitamin C and vitamin E during times of stress to keep our immunity strong so that stress does not lead to illness.

REJUVENATION FOODS TO EMPHASIZE

Vegetables

Dark green, leafy green, beets, cabbage.

Whole grains

All.

Fish

All.

Nuts

All.

Other foods

Nonfat yogurt, soybeans, tofu, white meat turkey, sunflower seeds, brewer's yeast.

SUPPLEMENTS INCREASED FROM REGULAR REJUVENATION INSURANCE

B-complex	100 mgs daily
Niacinamide	500 mgs daily
Vitamin B-6	50 mgs daily
Vitamin C	2000 mgs daily
Vitamin E	400 IUs daily
Calcium	1500 mgs daily
Magnesium	500 to 1000 mgs daily
Manganese	10 to 25 mgs daily
Zinc	30 mgs daily

THE EXERCISE FACTOR

Stress can cause fatigue. Do not allow this to be a reason not to exercise daily. During stressful periods exercise is all the more important, both in maintaining good health and in relieving stress. More than a few studies have concluded that rigorous activity can have an immediate diminishing effect on stress. I strongly recommend hatha yoga to anyone who seems to be constantly trying to cope with stress; for others, jabbing a punching bag or the violent swatting of a game of raquetball may offer some relief.

LIFESTYLE CONSIDERATIONS

Anyone who feels more than a little under stress should certainly take a good long look at his or her life and weigh the benefits of this lifestyle against the potential short-term and long-term effects on health. Some people need to rearrange their lives, rethink their priorities. Others need only to modify their responses to the world around them. Guided yoga and meditation can help, and ten to fifteen minutes per day of quiet relaxation, a daily minivacation, can benefit us all. Recent studies by a doctor in France found that listening to Gregorian chants in the background as often during the day as possible can be both energizing and relaxing (you need not go to a monastery to hear them; there are cassette tapes available); listening to Mozart tapes can also be helpful. Finally, at the risk of being obvious, a great way to diminish stress is to make sure that every single day of our lives we do something that is *fun.* For some of us this may mean discovering what fun is (what it used to be before we forgot); for others it simply means realizing that we are important enough to deserve to enjoy ourselves for at least part of each day.

Transient Ischemic Attack (TIA) Plan

IDENTIFICATION AND CAUSES

When blood flow is blocked in a localized area of the brain or fails to flow momentarily because of a heart rhythm abnormality, there are a variety of possible reactions in specific parts of the body. These are known as transient ischemic attacks. They are like miniature or mild pre-strokes, lasting less than twenty-four hours. (Any such attack lasting more than several hours is a stroke.) The reason they last only a few moments is that they are caused not by large blood clots but by tiny clots or spasming vessels, which usually cease their spasming after a short period of time. TIAs are not uncommon in persons over forty, especially (though not at all exclusively) those over 65, and may be the early warning signs of an impending stroke.

A TIA is often caused by the blockage (reduction in bore size) of the major arteries leading into the neck and the carotid arteries leading into the brain. This blockage or narrowing of arteries is often the same kind of arteriosclerosis-causing plaque that occurs in heart disease in response to high blood pressure, high cholesterol, and obesity, and in this case may be just as potentially fatal. Another possible cause is a tiny blood clot that may have shot out of the heart during an irregular rhythm—or in response to a damaged heart valve or any number of blood-clotting disorders—and into the brain, causing a blockage.

SYMPTOMS

One-sided vision loss is common in TIA; this usually corrects itself once the attack is over, though if a stroke follows it may become permanent. Dizziness, lightheadedness, double vision, neuritis or tingling of an extremity, numbness for no apparent reason, sudden fainting, or even just a passing confusion and temporary slurring of speech are all potential symptoms that require immediate medical attention. About ten percent of all transient ischemic attacks lead directly to a stroke.

TREATMENT

Since the symptoms of a TIA are similar to those associated with tumors, migraine headaches, and heart disease, a physician must first rule out these other illnesses to confirm that you did in fact have a transient ischemic attack. You'll then need to be checked for heart murmurs, have blood cholesterol measured, and undergo an EKG to check the heart rhythm. A CAT scan is also in order, as is a twenty-four-hour monitoring of the heart using a holter.

The most common and traditionally accepted therapy for the treatment of a TIA is aspirin—650 milligrams (two tablets twice a day). Cholesterol and blood pressure must be brought under control. See the High Cholesterol and High Blood Pressure Plans, and if you are overweight, see the Obesity Plan. For those with the most severe obstruction, surgery may be needed to replace those clotted arteries.

ANTI-TIA DIET

The Rejuvenation Diet plus the extra guidelines of the Anti-Cholesterol Diet (if needed), the Anti–High Blood Pressure Diet, and the Anti-Obesity Diet will cleanse your system. However, if you are on aspirin therapy for TIA, *do not use EPA capsules or vitamin E supplements,* as they may induce bleeding. On the other hand, if you are either allergic to aspirin or for some other reason are firmly against using it on a daily basis, you may replace it with EPA and vitamin E as suggested in the High-Cholesterol Plan. I do not, however, recommend this alternative over aspirin, and by all means discuss it with your doctor first.

THE EXERCISE FACTOR

See the High Cholesterol, High Blood Pressure, and Obesity Plans.

LIFESTYLE CONSIDERATIONS

See the High Cholesterol, High Blood Pressure, and Obesity Plans.

Ulcer Plan

IDENTIFICATION AND CAUSES

An ulcer is a hole in the lining of the stomach (called a peptic ulcer) or in the upper intestines (called a duodenal ulcer); both have the same symptoms and require the same treatment. About ten percent of all Americans, mostly men of all different ages, are afflicted at one time or another with an ulcer, though as women take on more stressful job and life situations, the risks are evening out among the sexes. Stress is certainly a major factor in the cause of ulcers, which according to current scientific theory is brought on by excess stomach acid and bacteria. Heredity may also play a role, though clearly no one is destined to get an ulcer simply because of a genetic predisposition toward them. Habitual users of aspirin and regular users of cortisone run a higher risk of contracting an ulcer and a lower chance of full recovery; and while there is no evidence that cigarette smoking is a cause of ulcers, it is clear that smoking will make an existing ulcer worse and may make healing take much longer. Some of the most recent studies on ulcers have linked excess saturated fats in the diet to the onset of duodenal ulcers, which are the most common kind.

SYMPTOMS

A searing stomach pain is the most common symptom, often occurring in the middle of the night. Unlike most stomach pain, an ulcer is relieved temporarily by food. Other symptoms include nausea, vomiting, unexplained weight loss, and back pain. If any of these symptoms persist for forty-eight to seventy-two hours, a medical examination is crucial. If untreated, an ulcer can perforate, causing a potentially fatal hemorrhage or peritonitis (infection).

TREATMENT

Through the right kind of therapy, ulcers can be completely healed. Until recently doctors used X rays to diagnose the presence of an ulcer, and this procedure missed as many as 30 percent of all ulcers. Now, however, by actually looking inside the stomach with an endoscope, doctors have virtually no chance of misdiagnosing. Medication can be helpful in treating an ulcer, especially the newer drugs such as Zantac and Tagamet, or carafate. Take them as per your doctor's prescription. Some doctors prescribe antacid liquid, which, in the case of treating ulcers, can be beneficial and outweigh their side effects (excess sodium, excess aluminum, and a tendency to be habit-forming), but they should be used only for the duration of the ulcer condition; and since antacids often deplete calcium, make sure you are taking a good calcium supplement daily (the standard rejuvenation dosage should be sufficient).

ANTI-ULCER DIET

Doctors once believed that milk was helpful in treating the symptoms of ulcers, and some even thought it was a cure. Until three years ago many doctors prescribed milk for patients with ulcers, believing it protected the stomach, neutralizing excess acid. And while milk as a treatment for ulcers still remains controversial, our most current information points to the conclusion that milk does not treat ulcers but instead may often worsen the condition. Milk may initially relieve discomfort but there is an acid rebound after about forty-five minutes, which floods the stomach with more acid than one would get from an identical amount of alcohol or coffee. Milk fat, as well as other saturated fats, is an irritant for most ulcers. While many physicians who specialize in the treatment of ulcers believe that no single food irritates all ulcers, most would agree—and my own observations confirm this—that there are certain suspect foods the ulcer patient should avoid until the ulcer is cured.

Coffee (even decaf), cocoa, tea, and chocolate are already eliminated in our Rejuvenation Diet, and there are some rejuvenation foods that the ulcer patient must add to his or her list of those to avoid.

REJUVENATION FOODS TO AVOID

High acid fruits

Apples, pears, pineapples, citrus fruits.

Alcoholic beverages (even in moderate amounts).

Vinegar and all spices and peppers

There are other foods which may help during the medical treatment of an ulcer. Some preliminary research suggests that fiber aids in the healing of an ulcerated stomach. Beta carotene, I have discovered, supports the integrity of mucus cell lining and growth that is necessary to protect the stomach lining, while vitamin C after each meal helps to build better intracellular "cement" and, in general, encourages healing.

It is now clear that food does not buffer the stomach, but rather, as part of the normal digestion process, food promotes the production of acid. So, whatever you eat, it is a good idea not to eat many small meals throughout the day, as was once commonly advised, but to opt for two or three moderate meals. Water, however, should be consumed as often as possible.

REJUVENATION FOODS TO EMPHASIZE

Vegetables

Leafy greens, dark greens, squash and other yellow and orange vegetables, cabbage and cabbage juice, potatoes, yams.

Fruits

Papayas, mangoes, pears, bananas, cantaloupes, cooked or dried apricots.

Whole grains

Oat bran, wheat bran.

SUPPLEMENTS INCREASED FROM REGULAR REJUVENATION INSURANCE

Beta carotene	25,000 IUs daily
Vitamin C	500 mgs after each meal

THE EXERCISE FACTOR

Exercise, especially hatha yoga, can play a major role in reducing stress and should therefore be a major part of anyone's recovery from an ulcer.

LIFESTYLE CONSIDERATIONS

Stop smoking to relieve your ulcer—if not for any of the many other health reasons—and start to do what is necessary to decrease stress in your life, be it biofeedback, time management, or simply pampering yourself, and immediately increase your life-span. See the Stress Plan for more information.

Vision Problem Plan

IDENTIFICATION AND CAUSES

The most common eye complaints I encounter with my patients are mostly generalized, such as eye fatigue, characterized by tiredness of the eyes and problems in reading, fluctuating vision, photophobia (extreme sensitivity to light), weak eye muscles, excess watering of the eyes, redness, burning, and recurring eye infections. Many believe these problems are the direct result of getting older, but this is not necessarily so. Other, more specific common eye disorders include detached retina, ulcers of the eye, nearsightedness (myopia), night blindness, detachment of the retinal nerve-head (retina pigmentosum), and glaucoma, a major vision problem for those over forty, characterized by high internal fluid pressure in the eye.

There are many potential factors contributing to all of these conditions, including heredity, misuse (such as reading for many years in poor light), or lack of use of eye muscles; but more and more evidence is also mounting which links eye disorders to specific foods in the diet. Animal fats, refined sugars and refined carbohydrates, excess salt, and, in general, heavily processed foods change the viscosity of fluid within the eye globe, changing the focal length of the eye's refraction and adversely affecting vision. Excess refined sugars, it has been recently suggested, deplete calcium from the elastic cells in the whites of the eyes. This can cause the eye to stretch out of its particular shape, changing the proper lens/camera effect. Excess refined sugars also deplete chromium which is necessary for good eye focusing.

Other recent findings point to a substantial influence of emotions on vision. Farsighted people, for example, tend to be emotionally farsighted; that is, they are often angry and have problems emotionally focusing on people or situations. Nearsighted people are often perfectionists, driven, compulsive; they are disinterested with anything beyond their immediate parameters, which is often as far as their eyes can clearly see. For further reading on the emotional-visual connection, see the Recommended Reading section.

SYMPTOMS

The symptoms of vision disorders are usually very noticeable and include anything from soreness to extreme eye pain; some symptoms, however, may be somewhat misleading. You may blame your boredom with the book you're reading if you get sleepy quickly while reading, when in fact it may be the result of a lack of visual fitness and a significant hint to get your eyes checked. Anyone over forty should have his or her eyes checked at least every two years or upon noticing any symptoms.

TREATMENT

Consider undergoing visual therapy under the guidance of a trained optometric specialist called a behavioral optometrist, found commonly at optometric schools. Regular optometrists can sometimes treat a disorder with eye exercises but may also determine that prescription lenses are needed. Opthalmologists and MDs will also prescribe laser therapy, or even surgery when needed. Always make sure to rule out dietary and emotional causes before allowing your doctor to prescribe glasses or eye surgery, and if necessary, get a second opinion. Make sure you are checked for glaucoma. Surgery or lasers can treat it, but left untreated, glaucoma is a common cause of blindness.

ANTI–VISION DISORDER DIET

The "good-vision" nutrients are vitamins A, B-complex, C, and E, the mineral zinc, and the essential fatty acid omega-3. Lack of vitamin A is associated with eye fatigue, light sensitivity (or photophobia), and recurring eye infections. Poor color vision may often be reversed with adequate B-2, and B-complex may be all that is needed to treat bloodshot eyes, eye muscle weakness, eyelid itch, and easy eye watering. In the case of retinal nerve hemorrhages, vitamins A, C, and E, as well as zinc and omega-3 have all been found to help. Some eye doctors also believe that vitamin E helps to treat detached retina; often they also find that weak eye muscles are improved with an increased dosage of vitamin E. Ulcers of the cornea seem to respond to B-complex, vitamin C, and increased total body protein. Night blindness has been found to respond to vitamin A, niacin, riboflavin, and zinc. And while there is no known cure for retinosa pigmentosa—a slowly failing retina and vision—vitamin A, vitamin E, lecithin, and omega-3 have helped to slow deterioration and improve vision for my patients and those of other doctors. Nearsightedness may be improved by simply cutting out refined sugars, refined carbohydrates, and caffeine; other eye disorders may be relieved just by cutting out excess saturated fat.

REJUVENATION FOODS TO EMPHASIZE

All fish

Fruits

Citrus fruits, papaya.

Vegetables

Carrots, yams.

All whole grains

All soy products

Seeds

Pumpkin seeds.

For corneal ulcers

Increase protein 30 percent above regular rejuvenation levels.*

SUPPLEMENTS INCREASED FROM REGULAR REJUVENATION INSURANCE

For detached retina

Vitamin E: 400 to 600 IUs daily.

For corneal ulcers

Vitamin C: 4000 to 6000 mgs daily.

For night blindness

Beta carotene: 10,000 IUs daily; niacin: 100 mgs daily; riboflavin: 30 to 50 mgs daily; zinc: 30 mgs daily.

*Make absolutely sure to get it from low-fat sources in order to keep fat at 15 to 20 percent of calories.

For retinosa pigmentosa

Beta carotene: 25,000 IUs daily; EPA capsules: 300 mgs daily.

THE EXERCISE FACTOR

Without eye exercise you can forget about good visual fitness. Like any other part of the body, lack of use is abuse. Here are some easy and very helpful eye exercises I use with my patients:

1. Focus on the tip of the nose, crossing your eyes until tears form, then close eyes, relax, and open them. Do four times a day for as long as possible.
2. Rapidly shift eye focus from near objects to far objects. Do this four times a day, two to four minutes each time. (If you do tedious, short vision work, you will find this particularly relaxing, especially if you do it during a break on the job.)
3. Hold a finger well extended and focus eyes on that finger, slowly bring the finger toward your nose, keeping both eyes on the finger so that eyes cross; bring the finger to the nose, close eyes, then remove finger. Do four times a day, ten each time.
4. Blink eyes rapidly while shifting eye focus from near to far, near to far. Do four times a day, one minute each time.

LIFESTYLE CONSIDERATIONS

If negative emotions and destructive perceptions can cause eye disorders, we have yet another reason to consider the advice in Chapter 6 and the Stress Plan.

Recommended Reading

Adams, Catherine F. *Nutritive Value of American Foods,* U.S. Department of Agriculture, 1975.

Bailey, Covert. *Fit or Fat?* Boston: Houghton Mifflin Co., 1978.

Banik, Allen E. *Your Water and Your Health.* Rev. ed. New Canaan, CT: Keats Publishing, 1981.

Biermann, June, and Barbara Toohey. *The Diabetic's Total Health Book.* Los Angeles: Jeremy P. Tarcher, 1980.

Bland, Jeffrey. *Your Health Under Siege: Using Nutrition to Fight Back.* Battleboro, VT: Stephen Greene Press, 1981.

______. ed, *Medical Applications of Clinical Nutrition.* New Canaan, CT: Keats Publishing, 1983.

______. *The Nutritional Supplement Analysis Laboratory of the Linus Pauling Institute of Science and Medicine.* Palo Alto, CA, 1984.

Braly, James. *Dr. Braly's Optimum Health Program.* New York: Laura Tarbet Times Books, 1985.

Branden, Nathaniel. *Honoring the Self.* Los Angeles: Jeremy P. Tarcher, 1983.

Brewster, Letitia, and Michael Jacobson. *The Changing American Diet.* Washington, DC: Center for Science in the Public Interest, 1983.

Burns, David D. *Feeling Good, The New Mood Therapy.* New York: New American Library, 1980.

Calabrese, Edward J. *Healthy Living in an Unhealthy World.* New York: Simon and Schuster, 1984.

Cheraskin, E., and W. M. Ringsdorf Jr., with Arlene Brecher. *Psychodietetics: Food as the Key to Emotional Health.* New York: Stein and Day, 1974.

Chopra, Depok. *Creating Health.* New York: Vantage, 1985.

Cousins, Norman. *Anatomy of an Illness as Perceived by the Patient: Reflections on Healing and Regeneration.* New York: Bantam, 1981.

Dadd, Debra L. *The Nontoxic Home.* Los Angeles: Jeremy P. Tarcher, 1986.

Dufty, William. *Sugar Blues.* Philadelphia: Chilton Book Company, 1975.

Fitch, Albert J., ed. *The Household Pollutants Guide.* New York: Anchor Books, Center for Science in the Public Interest, 1978.

Fredrick, Carlton. *Eating Right for You.* New York: Grosset and Dunlap, 1972.

———. *Dr. Carlton Frederick's New and Complete Nutritional Handbook.* Huntington Beach, CA: International Institute of Natural Health Sciences, 1976.

———. *Arthritis: Don't Learn to Live with It.* New York: Grosset and Dunlap, 1981.

Fries, James F. *Arthritis: A Comprehensive Guide.* Reading, MA: Addison-Wesley, 1979.

Fuchs, Nan Kathryn. *The Nutrition Detective.* Los Angeles: Jeremy P. Tarcher, 1985.

Galloway, Jeff. *Galloway's Book on Running.* Bolinas, CA: Shalter Publications, 1984.

Gold, Mark S. *Good News About Depression.* Knightstown, IN: Bookmark Books, Inc., 1986.

Goodhard, Robert S., and Maurice E. Shils, eds. *Modern Nutrition in Health and Disease,* 6th ed. Philadelphia: Lea & Febiger, 1980.

Hausman, Patricia. *Jack Sprat's Legacy: The Science and Politics of Fat and Cholesterol.* New York: Richard Marek Publishers, 1981.

———. *The Right Dose.* Emmaus, PA: Rodale Press, 1987.

Hewitt, Jean. *The New York Times New Natural Foods Cookbook.* New York: Avon, 1983.

Hunter, Beatrice Trum. *Fact/Book on Food Additives and Your Health.* New Canaan, CT: Keats Publishing, 1972.

International Vitamin A Consultative Group (IVACG). *Guidelines for the Eradication of Vitamin A Deficiency and Xerophthalmia.* New York: 1976.

Kirschmann, John D. *Nutrition Almanac.* New York: McGraw-Hill, 1979.

Kordel, L. *Health Through Nutrition.* New York: MacFadden-Bartell, 1971.

Kushi, Michio, and Alex Jack. *The Cancer Prevention Diet.* New York: St. Martin's Press, 1983.

Lappe, Frances M. *Diet for a Small Planet.* 10th Anniversary Edition. New York: Ballantine, 1982.

Lawrence, Ron, and Sandra Rosenzweig. *Going the Distance: The Right Way to Exercise for People Over Forty.* Los Angeles: Jeremy P. Tarcher, 1987.

Levin, Alan S., and Merla Zellerbach. *The Type 1/Type 2 Allergy Relief Program.* Los Angeles: Jeremy P. Tarcher, 1983.

Mindell, Earl. *Earl Mindell's Pill Bible.* New York: Bantam Books, 1984.

National Research Council. *Recommended Dietary Allowances.* 8th ed., revised. Washington, DC: National Academy of Sciences, 1973.

Passwater, Richard A. *Super Nutrition.* New York: Dial, 1975.

Pauling, Linus. *Vitamin C and the Common Cold.* New York: Bantam Books, 1971.

Pritikin, Nathan. *The Pritikin Permanent Weight-Loss Manual.* New York: Grosset and Dunlap, 1981.

Rodale, J. I. *The Complete Book of Minerals for Health.* 4th ed. Emmaus, PA: Rodale Books, 1976.

Rosenberg, Harold, and A. N. Feldzman. *Doctor's Book of Vitamin Therapy: Megavitamins for Health.* New York: Putnam, 1974.

Ruthe, Eshleman, and Mary Winston, comps. *The American Heart Association Cookbook.* New York: Ballantine, 1973.

Saifer, Phyllis, and Merla Zellerbach. *Detox.* Los Angeles: Jeremy P. Tarcher, 1984.

Sehnert, Keith W., with Howard Eisenberg. *How To Be Your Own Doctor.* New York: Grosset and Dunlap, 1975.

Selye, Hans. *Stress Without Distress.* New York: New American Library, 1974.

Tatker, Brad. *Better Health Through Natural Living.* New York: McGraw-Hill, 1985.

U.S. Senate. Select Committee on Nutrition and Human Needs. *National*

Nutritional Policy: Nutrition and the Consumer II. Washington, DC: U.S. Government Printing Office, 1974.

The Walking Magazine, 711 Boylston St., Boston, MA 02116.

Williams, Roger J. *Nutrition Against Disease.* New York: Pitman Publishers, 1971.

Index